H (

NON-SMOKING KIDS

HOW TO

RAISE

NON-SMOKING

KIDS

DR. NEIL IZENBERG

WITH ROBERT P. LIBBON

BYRON PREISS MULTIMEDIA COMPANY, INC.

NEW YORK

POCKET BOOKS

New York London Toronto Sydney Tokyo Singapore

An Original Publication of Pocket Books

Pocket Books, a division of Simon & Schuster Inc.
1230 Avenue of the Americas, New York, NY 10020

Byron Preiss Multimedia Company, Inc.
24 West 25th Street
New York, New York 10010

The Byron Preiss Multimedia World Wide Web Site Address is:
http://www.byronpreiss.com

ISBN 0-671-01170-7

First Pocket Books paperback printing November 1997

10 9 8 7 6 5 4 3 2 1

Senior Editor: Dinah Dunn
Editorial Assistant: Cindy Schwalb
Cover design: Stephen Jablonoski
Interior design: Jessica Shatan

Printed in the U.S.A.

CONTENTS

Foreword   **vii**

Introduction   **1**

What Are Kids Thinking?   **8**

Preparing Your Kids for the Pressure to Smoke   **13**

Why Kids Smoke—and What You Can Do   **21**
  Smoking Is Accepted Within the Family   **21**
  Peer Pressure: "Everyone's Doing It"   **23**
  The Search for Independence and Adulthood   **28**
  The Romance of Risk and Rebellion: Too Cool to Care   **29**
  Chilling Out: Smoking as Relief   **34**

What if Your Kids Smoke Anyway?   **36**

Combating Marketing and Myth   **40**

Combating the Compulsion to Smoke   **57**

A Quiz for You and Your Kids   **62**

A Few Responses to Kids' Questions about Smoking   **75**

The History of Tobacco in American Culture   **82**

Cessation Methods   **93**

Resources   **99**

FOREWORD

BY STUART M. COPPERMAN M.D. /F.A.A.P.

My sixteen-year-old patient told me she was angry at her boyfriend. "Why?" I asked. She responded, "Because he just started smoking!" I said, "Melissa, you've been smoking since you were twelve." She replied, "Yes, but I didn't know any better then. He's old enough and smart enough to know not to start at seventeen."

Melissa was right. The vast majority of smokers start before they are thirteen years old. When they get "smart enough" to want to quit, they find to their dismay that they are hooked. That is why this book, with techniques both innovative as well as tried and true, is so appropriate for parents of preteens. Using facts, common sense, and a good sprinkling of humor, the text gives concerned parents (as we all should be, since silence is acceptance) a smorgasbord of methods to help keep their child from using tobacco.

Why do parents need to be involved? We are fighting an uphill battle against an industry that entices 3,000 teenagers a day to start smoking, who become replacement smokers for those who are able to quit and for those who die. The tobacco

industry is so successful that, despite all the frightening medical facts and scare tactics we can muster, the incidence of
smoking cigarettes among eighth graders had increased 50
percent in the past five years, from 14 percent to 21 percent.
And it doesn't just end with tobacco use—studies show that
the use of cigarettes by children yields a five-fold increase in
the likelihood of other future addictive behavior. In order to
stop a new generation from picking up that first cigarette, we
must adjust our tactics.

As a pediatrician who has been active in the battle to keep
kids from starting to smoke for over thirty years, I can tell you
why I am concerned. Smoking will cause the premature death
of more than five million Americans who are now under eighteen years old. Cigarettes maim and kill, not just through
lung cancer and emphysema, but through fires, increased incidence of automobile accidents among smokers, and other
tragedies.

Why are cigarettes so popular with kids despite all of the
diseases linked to their usage? They are inexpensive, available,
and attractive—therefore, the three areas we need to combat.
In 1993, the tobacco industry spent over $6 billion on adver-
tising, promotions, sports, and cultural events to make cigarettes more "cool." Was it effective? And how. Before Joe
Camel appeared, only three percent of kids smoked Camels.
After that deluge of advertising, now 25 percent smoke them.
Are cigarettes available? You bet! Ninety percent of kids are
not stopped when they tried to buy cigarettes from vending
machines. At least 50 percent of kids who try can buy cigarettes in stores, despite laws to the contrary.

While the FDA is limiting tobacco access and advertising,
a new approach is still needed to make non-smoking "cool"

and smoking just dumb and dumber. *How to Raise Non-Smoking Kids* gives parents ways at home to keep their children from starting to smoke, such as setting a good example by not smoking, keeping lines of discussion open, and providing good answers to difficult questions.

On a national level, the American Academy of Pediatrics had established the "Tobacco Free Generation," employing tactics such as positive role models from entertainment and sports, peer identification, "NicoTeams," poster contests, and media coverage to help attain the elusive "Smoke Free Society."

Schools can help. In the elementary schools, part of the curriculum in math, history, social studies, economics, as well as health, should include a discussion about tobacco. Students who see the behavior modification techniques of the tobacco advertisers may be less likely to fall for them. Students who see tobacco use as $3-5/a day or $1500/a year literally going up in smoke may decide to save the money for car insurance, instead. Schools can set up the equivalent of the old "G.O. Cards" for certified non-smokers to get discounts at local pizza parlors, fast-food stores, bowling alleys, computer stores, driving ranges, skating rinks, stationery stores, etc., to demonstrate the social (and economic) value of non-smoking. All schools should be totally smoke-free, including teachers' lounges and maintenance areas.

Parents can ask their children's doctors to get involved in the schools. For example, pediatricians and pediatric residents nationwide are using of their free time to go into schools to discuss the good things about being a non-smoker. College students are being trained to speak to high-school kids. This chain could extend until we eventually have junior-high stu-

dents going into the elementary schools to talk about the stu-
pidity of smoking. Involved parents can get this started in
their school districts

The American Medical Association (AMA) is fighting
smoke with fire! They have created a cartoon character, the
Extingisher, to defeat Joe Camel, Kool Penguins, and
Marlboro Cowboys on their own battlefields. Once a smoker
near death, the Extingisher's superpowers come from the heal-
ing efforts of a female physician, Dr. Nola Know. Together,
they go off to "kick butts" wherever they find them. Working
with *Scholastic News*, the AMA is enrolling kids in a nationwide contest in which they sign pledges to be "tobacco free"
and explain how they intend to help in the fight against
smoking.

How to Raise Non-Smoking Kids serves a valuable function in
enlisting the most important advocacy group for children—
parents—in the battle to save lives and to enhance the quality
of lives. Even parents who smoke can join in this effort. It's a
rare adult smoker who would wish his or her habit on a
twelve-year-old. This is not an "us versus them" battle, but an
effort to create a Tobacco Free Generation—a campaign we
can all support. This book will help.

                                Stuart M. Copperman, M.D., F.A.A.P.

*Dr. Copperman is president of the Nassau County (New York)
Pediatric Society, a media representative for the American Academy of
Pediatrics, and founder and coordinator of their Tobacco Free
Generation campaign. He is in private practice of pediatrics and ado-
lescent medicine in Merrick, New York.*

INTRODUCTION

On June 20, 1997, representatives from the tobacco industry reached a potentially historic settlement with the attorneys general of thirty-nine states, a settlement that, even if ratified without dramatic alteration, would make vast changes in the regulation and marketing of tobacco products. In addition to providing an industry fund to compensate states for the health costs of smoking-induced diseases, the tobacco companies agreed to

- permanently retire the Marlboro Man and Joe Camel, two notorious advertising icons which anti-smoking activists blame for a huge increase in smoking by kids. In addition, the tobacco companies agreed to stop using human and cartoon characters in their advertisements, placing tobacco products in movies and on television, sponsoring sporting events, and giving away merchandise bearing cigarette logos

- reduce teenage smoking by 60 percent in ten years, with milestones to be met along the way and monetary penalties for unmet goals

- shell out at least $500 million on anti-smoking messages designed specifically to keep teenagers from smoking

- fund both anti-smoking public education campaigns and smoking cessation programs.

Parents around the country celebrated the end of the tobacco industry's concerted and highly successful effort to entice children and teenagers to smoke, and breathed a sigh of relief. At last, their kids were safe from tobacco.

Not.

If you think this agreement—or, indeed, any negotiated agreement with tobacco companies—will keep your kid from smoking, think again. Ask yourself why the tobacco companies bought into this settlement. They had no choice? They were facing crippling class action lawsuits? They were hon-

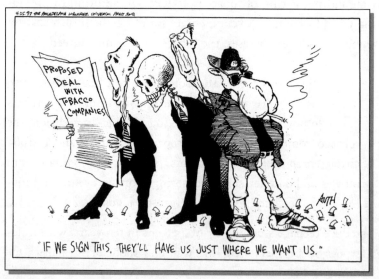

Tony Auth/Universal Press Syndicate

estly concerned with the welfare of the country's children? They honestly intend to spearhead a drive to reduce teenage smoking?

Nope. They signed off on this agreement because they, more than anyone else in this country, understand why people start to smoke. Their livelihoods depend upon people smoking. Their corporate survival depends on attracting new smokers to replace those who manage to quit and those who finally die. The tobacco companies agreed to this settlement because they know that despite the health-care provisions, despite the ban on certain types of advertising, despite aid to cessation and prevention programs, the settlement fails to address the most important issue: Why kids want to smoke.

Tobacco companies know that they'll be able to market their product as long as smoking has cultural and psychological merit. Banning advertising that features hip characters and role models takes an important weapon out of the tobacco industry's arsenal—but tobacco companies have other weapons. Ban role models who exemplify independence, strength, beauty, and cool? Wait for the billboards with slogans that are soothing, bold, beautiful, or stark. Eliminate product placement in movies and television and get rid of advertising in convenience stores? Watch for a new round of magazine advertisements: black pages featuring the name of a cigarette, a huge surgeon general's warning, and two words: "Adults Only." And if you think that type of advertisement will keep kids from smoking . . . well, you don't know kids.

Hoping that a simple settlement will keep kids from smoking is like believing that the 1954 Supreme Court decision in *Brown v. Board of Education* put an end to racism. Keeping your kids from picking up a cigarette takes more than an agreement signed by a bunch of attorneys general, a couple of anti-smoking lobbyists, and the multinational tobacco industry.

To illustrate the point, imagine a scenario much more restrictive than the settlement outlined above. All cigarette advertising is banned. Brand names of cigarettes are outlawed completely; instead, only a generic item known as the "Coffin Nail" is to be sold. All sales of Coffin Nails are to take place in government-regulated Quonset huts hidden inside deeply wooded compounds. Armed sentries restrict admission to those over eighteen years of age.

Smoking is allowed only in geodesic domes that purify and recirculate the same air within, so that no smoke ever leaves the unit. Once again, admission is monitored by armed guards who check each user's ages, and see to it that every smoker-user has signed the Smoker's Waiver of Health, Responsibility, and Liability. In addition, smoker-users must show proof of the ability to pay for his or her own health care should he or she fall victim to any smoking-related disease or disability. Should a smoker-user not have sufficient means, he or she must sign a voluntary euthanasia pledge, to be effected at the first signs of a smoking-related illness. Said euthanasia will be paid for by the taxes on all cigarettes.

As unlikely (one can only hope) as the above scenario seems, you'd think that this would finally put a lid on teenage smoking, right?

Wrong. While the draconian regime described above might result in a *reduction* in teen smoking, it would hardly eliminate it altogether. Instead, teenage smoking would simply go undercover, along with a huge black market of cigarette dealers, brand makers, and clandestine smoking dens.

Kids would still be able to smoke. What's worse, in many ways that scenario would make it *even cooler* to smoke than it is today.

This is what the tobacco industry has known for years: As long as there is a demand for a given commodity, there will be a market for it. Remember Prohibition? The legal marketplace for liquor was abolished, but the demand wasn't addressed. That gave us bootleggers, speakeasies, and a hugely successful and powerful new criminal class. The war on drugs? Arrest dealers, close off the borders, sever relations with countries that condone drug production, and what happens? With the demand left in place, new dealers spring up, new routes into the country develop, and offending countries make enough money to shrug off any international sanctions.

In order to seriously reduce kids' smoking, we have to address the adolescent demand for cigarettes. And when I say "we," I mean you—the parents.

If you think about it, *How to Raise Non-Smoking Kids* is a rather presumptuous title. Imagine a book entitled *How to Raise Doctors*, or more to the point, *How to Raise Non-Swearing Kids*. What are we after, anyway? Are we suggesting that you can groom your offspring to follow the patterns you'd like to see them adopt? Are there methods for raising vegetarian kids, jazz-loving kids, kids with great fadeaway jump shots?

Certainly not. Kids have ways of surprising us with their own preferences, their own goals and desires, their own choices. In fact, the search for independence is part of the essential struggle of adoloescence. About age twelve (give or take a couple years), kids who automatically accepted your view of the world, who seemed eager to please or at least get along, undergo a seemingly dramatic transformation. As they develop increasing physical and intellectual independence (and those complex hormones begin to kick in), early teens begin to question and challenge. And that's normal.

For most kids—the transition toward adulthood is relatively smooth and painless, just a few bumps here and there. Studies have shown that most teens still want to be like their parents and share their values. For others, those years are difficult—full of conflict, pain, and even danger to themselves. This stage, however temporary, can be a real challenge to parents.

Some kids turn in the opposite direction from their parents' preferences in a show of independence, or rebellion, or loyalty to their peers. Some will do things that seem designed just to earn the disapproval of their parents: from getting tattoos, to playing (or not playing) sports, to hanging out with the "wrong" crowd, and to listening to the "wrong" sorts of music. The list goes on. Some of these things are downright dangerous: climbing water towers or jumping on moving trains or elevators, breaking into buildings or into computers, riding skateboards or skates perilously in traffic, and drinking and smoking. Smoking for any of a number of reasons: to fit in, to feel or look older, to be cool, to lose weight (a big one for girls), to win hip merchandise, to seem tough, and to feel independent.

But smoking for most people isn't a one-time ritual, a youthful lark, or a milestone in adolescent development. It may appear to be a childish way to fit in, or to look tough, just as driving too fast or taking dares are childish. But there's a difference. As they become adults, teenagers discover that such dares, pranks, and stunts are no longer necessary to define them or to secure their place in society. But when teenagers realize that smoking isn't necessary, what they discover is that they can't stop. Their youthful habit has become a deadly addiction.

Smoking is a trap set for teenagers, one that advertises itself as a panacea for adolescent ills, the answer to any perceived shortcoming, any urgent need. Advertising, history, and cultural myth all contribute to the belief that tobacco is a solution, while hiding the fact that smoking is actually a life-threatening addiction. The immediacy of its dubious benefits masks long-term hazards that, for a twelve-year-old, are simply too distant to mean anything.

Studies show that very few smokers, only 10 percent, take up the habit as adults, because adults have the maturity and the foresight to see the idiocy of such a move. Studies show that for lifetime smokers, twelve years old was the average age that smoking began in earnest. Your job as parent is to give your kid the tools and attitudes needed to make it through adolescence without turning to tobacco.

How can you counter a multi-billion-dollar industry, political expediency, expert advertising, and a cultural history that glorifies tobacco use? You don't have access to the tobacco companies' marketing studies. You don't have direct access to Congress. You aren't as "cool" as Johnny Depp or Kate Moss. All you have is access to your kid.

But that's all you really need.

WHAT ARE KIDS THINKING?

Since 1965 every pack of cigarettes has come with a mandated warning from the surgeon general about the hazards of smoking, a warning that has both multiplied and grown more emphatic over the years. Pick up a pack of smokes today and you'll see one of the following:

- SURGEON GENERAL'S WARNING: Smoking Causes Lung Cancer, Heart Disease, Emphysema, and May Complicate Pregnancy;

- SURGEON GENERAL'S WARNING: Quitting Smoking Now Greatly Reduces Serious Risks to Your Health;

- SURGEON GENERAL'S WARNING: Smoking by Pregnant Women May Result in Fetal Injury, Premature Birth, and Low Birth Weight;

- SURGEON GENERAL'S WARNING: Cigarette Smoke Contains Carbon Monoxide.

What's more, for decades parents, teachers, and doctors have been preaching the evils of tobacco to children, telling them the cold, hard, nasty facts about smoking. And the result of this effort to educate and warn children? More than 90 percent of all smokers still begin smoking as teens and every year some 3,000 kids still start smoking.

Why?

For one thing, the above warnings don't say the same things to a kid as they do to adults. Here's a teen translation of the warnings:

- A STUFFY OLD GOVERNMENT DOCTOR SAYS: Smoking causes lung cancer, heart disease, and emphysema if you smoke for years and years, and doesn't necessarily complicate pregnancy, which isn't in my game plan right now anyway;

- A STUFFY OLD GOVERNMENT DOCTOR SAYS: I can quit anytime I want with no serious health consequences;

- A STUFFY OLD GOVERNMENT DOCTOR SAYS: Smoking by pregnant women may result in fetal injury, premature birth, and low birth weight, so if I ever think about getting pregnant I'll stop smoking;

- A STUFFY OLD GOVERNMENT DOCTOR SAYS: Smoking is like being in traffic.

Stack these warnings up against the following messages kids get about smoking from history, popular culture, advertising, and their peers:

- THE COOLEST GUY I KNOW SAYS: Smoking causes immediate acceptance into my crowd, pal;

- THE THINNEST GIRL IN MY CLASS SAYS: Smoking is a wonderful substitute for food;

- THE GUY WHO'S AS UNHAPPY AS I AM SAYS: Smoking greatly reduces my feeling of helplessness and relaxes me;

- THE HIPPEST STARS, MALE AND FEMALE, AT A MOVIE PREMIERE SAY: The sure sign of success is a monster cigar.

You get the picture. The marked increase in teenage smoking over the past decades shows that the traditional method of discouraging smoking—education coupled with scare tactics—simply isn't effective. Teenagers know that smoking is bad for them. They've seen the pictures of lungs taken during autopsies of smokers. They've heard the statistics. Facts, although important, don't attack the heart of the problem. Kids don't start smoking because they want to be addicted, or because it ruins them for sports, discolors their teeth, and makes them smell rotten. Nor do they particularly care if it will kill them some day; the progressive effects of smoking are too distant for youngsters who've only been alive a dozen or so years, and who can't grasp the fact of their own mortality. Facts, no matter how clear and intimidating, are overshadowed by desire. It's a choice driven by emotion, and in order to enable kids to make a different choice, you have to address the emotion.

Clearly, a different approach is needed, one that not only educates kids about smoking but attacks the question of smoking in important ways by

- preempting the particular reasons why teenagers start to smoke,

- exploding the myths that surround smoking,

- exposing the ingenious methods tobacco merchants use to attract teenagers,

- emphasizing not the negative aspects of smoking, but the positive benefits of a non-smoking life: good health, physical fitness, and more disposable income,

- reinforcing what a large percentage of the teenage population already know: not smoking is cool.

Preparing kids for the onslaught of pro-smoking messages, giving them the tools to decide against smoking, and redefining "cool" as the province of the non-smoker, then, are the broad elements in raising a non-smoking kid.

As we look at the concrete steps you can take to raise a non-smoking kid, you'll discover one essential theme running throughout: communication. Oh, you can watch your kid like a hawk, make all the rules you want, and pound the medical statistics into your kid's head. Unless you know how to communicate, however, none of it will be worth a damn. And communicating doesn't mean lecturing or interrogating or punishing, although that is sometimes appropriate. Communicating means talking and listening to your kid in order to understand each other. One teenager we talked with, Ilana, said, "If parents really don't want their kids to smoke, they should stop yelling so much. They should talk to them and then let them make the decision. I see it all the time—the more the parents yell, the more and more their kids rebel."

After all, raising a non-smoking kid doesn't involve brainwashing, but rather showing him or her how to make independent decisions, how to think critically. It means replacing the attraction of smoking with positive non-smoking images and activities. It means giving support, and helping to build a healthy sense of self-worth and self-esteem. It means showing your child how to question, how to examine, how to learn— and for many parents, it means discovering these things themselves. These are the tools that will help guide kids through adolescence—indeed, through their entire lives—without falling victim to false promises, self-doubt, and the pressure to needlessly conform.

PREPARING YOUR KIDS FOR THE PRESSURE TO SMOKE

You've got about twelve years before your child becomes the active target of tobacco advertising and becomes acutely vulnerable to cultural and societal pressure to smoke. Although twelve is the average age, much younger kids are aware of tobacco advertising and themes.

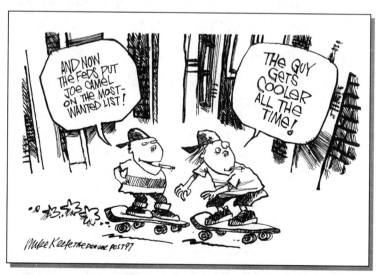

Mike Keefe/*The Denver Post*/dePiXion Studios, Inc.

Kids can hit adolescence with one of three attitudes: pro-tobacco, tobacco-neutral, or anti-tobacco. And while there are no guarantees as to the outcome—kids will continue to confound the predictions of us adults—you can set attitudes and habits in the home that when the time comes will help head off your kid's temptation to smoke.

Here are some things you can do before your kid reaches adolescence:

1. Hmmm . . . let's see . . . how about you not smoking? Now there's a good idea. If you happen to smoke now, stop. Even if you don't have any kids but think you might want to have children someday and you smoke now, stop. Safeguarding your kids from smoking starts with your not smoking. One teenage smoker, Denise, put it well, "Both my parents are smokers. With all the second-hand smoke I inhale, anything I do is superfluous." And just in case some of you moms-to-be are thinking of putting off quitting until your kid is born, remember that a pregnant woman who smokes is smoking for two. Smoking during pregnancy

- deprives the baby of oxygen,

- increases the likelihood that your baby will have a lower birth weight than others,

- exposes your baby to a greater range of health complications than the babies of non-smokers, such as being four times more likely to get cancer under the age of six,

- increases the likelihood that your child will be hyperactive or learning disabled.

2. If you are an ex-smoker, be prepared to one day explain why you started and, most importantly, why you stopped. Emphasize

how your life has changed for the better since quitting: how much money you've saved, how much easier it is to breathe, how good you feel and look and even smell.

3. Set clear rules about smoking in the home and enforce them. If it means Aunt Virginia doesn't come over anymore, so be it. Your kid must realize that your stand on smoking is firm.

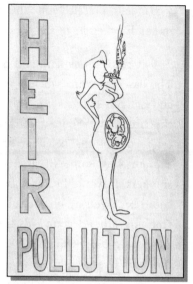

4. Let your kid know why you have set such rules. A first-grader might not be

Steve Korin, Mark Twain Jr. High School 239, Brooklyn, N.Y. © 1991.

able to grasp the progressive aspects of smoking, but he can certainly understand that tobacco is listed as a "Bad Thing," and that smokers smell bad, look bad, and feel bad.

5. Get your kid involved in activities that preclude smoking, and thereby avoid activities that encourage or condone it. Who do you think stands the better chance of avoiding tobacco as a teen: a physically active kid who shares something like hiking or swimming with friends and relatives, or an inactive kid whose idea of physical and mental involvement is locating the remote control while Cousin Lucky looks for his lighter?

6. Explain to children as young as two years old how the reality of smoking contrasts with images in popular culture. It probably won't have much effect on your kid, but it gives you

a chance to practice your anti-smoking spiel, which will come in handy when he or she gets older.

7. Get ready to explain and defend the stupid things you do. The day may come when your kid decides to have a cigarette, and defends it by saying something like "Well, you drink all the time," or "You eat too much red meat!" And since you can't control the behavior of others, you should be able to explain why some (if any) of your friends or relatives are smokers. It would be a nice bonus if those friends and relatives could back you up on the subject, not only by refraining from smoking around your kids but by explaining why they wish they could quit, why they can't (or won't), and how much better their lives would be without tobacco. (Naturally, if their reasons for smoking includes "It makes me feel cool," you're better off not enlisting their help.)

8. Know what you're talking about. When your kid asks why smoking is bad, you don't want to have to answer: "Uhhhh . . . because." In the back of this book are a list of organizations that can provide you with recent information about the dangers of smoking. Keep up on the latest tobacco news, and include your kid in the process when he or she is old enough. Better you find out together what's happening than for you to become Joe Lecturer.

A word about advocacy: It's terribly tempting to make the case against smoking by inflating figures ("Every 1.5 seconds a smoker dies"), attributing additional unpleasant side effects ("Secondary cigarette smoke causes insanity in household pets"), or turning it into a religious issue ("Smokers are evil demons who someday will burn just like their cigarettes"). Not only is this a dubious tactic to use on young kids—who might end up being terrified of smokers and their pets—but it tends to backfire as your kid realizes your deception.

When talking to your kid about smoking, it is essential that you communicate the facts, and the facts alone. There is no need for invention; the truth itself is bad enough. Embellishment, distortion, and deceit are the weapons of the tobacco industry. Resorting to them in the belief that the end (a non-smoking kid) justifies the means (being dishonest about the effects of smoking) is a fatal temptation. As soon as a kid sees that you have been less than honest in talking about smoking, you cease to be a beacon of truth and become just another bore.

A few non-smoking groups make this mistake in a misguided (if understandable) attempt to persuade others of their position. Taking preliminary and often vague scientific findings, they draw unsupported opinions from inconclusive stud-

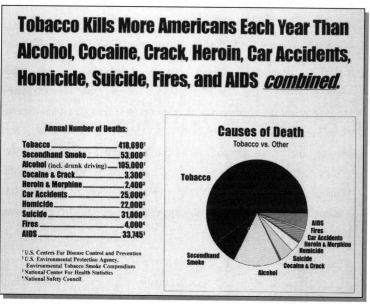

Smokefree Educational Services, Inc., NY, NY.

ies. This only throws their own motives and integrity into question, and allows both smokers and smoker-wanna-bes a loophole: *Sure, the tobacco giants distort the facts, but so does the anti-smoking lobby, and so do my parents. So until an unbiased source of information comes along, I think I'll have a cigarette.*

9. Read with your kid, watch television with your kid, go to the movies with your kid, and compare what you see with what you know about the everyday world. For example:

•Watch a heavy-smoking hero running away from the bad guys. Does he end up wheezing and coughing when he finally escapes (or gets captured)? Wouldn't he be more likely to escape his pursuers if he had healthy lungs?

•Talk about what you don't see and hear. When the camera moves in on two smokers whispering sweet nothings to one another, do you hear the little wheeze so common to daily smokers? Does either of them suddenly break out into a hacking fit? Why not?

•See a movie like *The Maltese Falcon*, in which Humphrey Bogart portrays tough, savvy, cigarette-rolling private detective Sam Spade. Check out how many of the characters smoke, and then ask yourself what happened not to the characters who look so good smoking, but to the actors. Humphrey Bogart died at fifty-seven of cancer of the esophagus and Mary Astor died of emphysema, as did director John Huston.

•Expose your kid to role models who don't smoke. There are plenty of celebrities and sports figures who have taken a stand against tobacco.

As you can see, the most important way you can prepare to deal with smoking is by establishing good communication with your kid. The more you talk to your kid about any important subject, the better chance you have of staying close when things get tough. Make it part of your daily routine to just sit around and talk with (not lecture) your kid. Communication, after all, isn't just talking but knowing when to be an adviser, when to be a storyteller, when to be an authoritarian—and when to just shut up and be a listener. It's a fine line to walk. Usually it's easier to say what not to do.

- Don't overreact.

- Don't use sarcasm or ridicule.

- Don't avoid subjects because you might find them uncomfortable.

- Don't force your kid to talk on your terms and on your time.

- Don't interrogate.

- Don't show disrespect, even if you find your kid's opinions unformed and illogical.

- Don't assume that the same things that worked with one kid will necessarily be appropriate to another.

There are some of the things you can do.

- Let them know that their hopes, dreams, day-to-day activities, and difficulties are important to you. Participate wherever possible. Share activities with your kid—even if it's just sitting around humming.

- Reward and encourage your kid when she reaches a goal, takes responsibility, asks questions, and even questions answers.

- Be ready to listen when your kid wants to talk. If there's no way you can sit down at the moment, let your kid know why and schedule a time when you can talk.

- Your kid might have kid problems, but to him they're earth-shaking dilemmas. Treat them as seriously as your kid does.

- Take an active interest in your kid's schoolwork. You're the most important influence in your kid's life. If you're not interested, how is your kid going to be?

- Arm your child with feelings of self-confidence and self-worth. That's a life-long process which begins way before adolescence. What do self-confidence and self-worth have to do with smoking? Everything. With much of the advertising about smoking aimed subtly at rebellion and being cool and one of the major struggles of adolescence being the push for independence, the combination can be lethal. Kids who feel belittled or undervalued at home, who are bound in and overly controlled, will seek to escape one way or another. It's no coincidence that the parents who run the "tightest ship," who are the most authoritarian and punitive, often have the most rebellious teens.

Among the most important tasks of parents is to teach their kids the confidence and self skills to master the world on their own, and not only on command. Loving, consistent, and firm discipline is an important part of growing up, but discipline needs to be learned from within or it just breaks down.

WHY KIDS SMOKE—AND WHAT YOU CAN DO

Smoking Is Accepted Within the Family

In 1968, following an FCC ruling that required TV stations who carried tobacco commercials to provide free time for anti-smoking "commercials," powerful anti-smoking ads began to appear. One of the most memorable featured a small boy mimicking his father's actions as they spent some relaxed "quality time" together: throwing a rock across a pond, picking a blade of grass, sitting up against a tree . . . and reaching for a pack of cigarettes. The message was clear: like father, like son. (In fact, it was the potency of this and other anti-smoking commercials that convinced tobacco companies to agree to a ban on broadcast advertisment of their products; it meant the end of anti-smoking ads as well.)

A teenager's susceptibility to the lure of tobacco has a lot to do with the attitudes and values present in the home. Obviously, a kid whose parents smoke might very well adopt the attitude that smoking is an acceptable habit. I say "might very well" because some kids actually find their parents' hacking and coughing and odor as a turn-off. Go figure. But more typical is the statement of one long-time smoker: "I have a lot of people in my family who smoke and, of course, at the time that they were smoking and I had started, none of them were dying of it yet."

Take a look at what some kids have to say about smoking in the home, and see if you can guess what they all have in common:

"Smoking is OK if you're old enough; my parents smoke."

"Smoking is OK until you want to have kids. Then you can just stop, like my parents."

"My Uncle Ted smoked, and he lived until he was ninety-four."

"My mom smoked when I was growing up, and it never bothered me."

Easy, right? They're all smokers.

What you can do: Examine your own attitudes, not just about tobacco, but about other substances as well.

- Do you sigh nostalgically when the subject of marijuana comes up?

- Do you stagger into the house at the end of a day, saying, "I need a drink"?

- Do you often say things like, "I'm worthless until I have that first cup of coffee to get me going?"

These sort of statements teach kids that for every human weakness or setback, there's a substance to make it easier— alcohol, tobacco, caffeine, marijuana, and so on. That's hardly the attitude that you, as your child's first and most influential role model, should be conveying. What your kid needs to learn by your example is that most problems are solved by compassion, honesty, love and a little hard work—none of which come prepackaged in a bottle, weed, bean, or grain.

Peer Pressure: "Everyone's Doing It"

We all know how most kids respond to the time-honored parental question, "If everyone jumped off the Brooklyn Bridge, would you?" Your kid averts his eyes, adopts a posture somewhere between tolerance and exasperation, and mechanically provides the right answer: "No." But when it comes to smoking, a more appropriate version of the question might be, "If everyone jumped off the Brooklyn Bridge and it took forty years to hit the water, would you?" Every day some 3,000 kids answer "yes" to that question when they light up for the first time—and the second and the third.

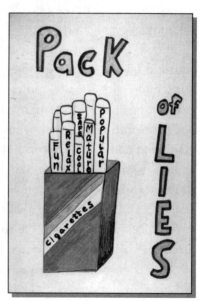

Caheim Drake, P. S. 112, Bronx, N.Y. © 1991. Smokefree Educational Services, Inc., NY, NY.

The search for social acceptance is a powerful motivator, especially as kids begin the transition into adulthood. Parental wisdom and authority, so effective in the past in guiding and protecting children, suddenly has strong, often overwhelming competition. You've managed to keep a smoke-free household, even convinced your brother-in-law to stop smoking, and let your kids know that non-smokers live the coolest lives—and one day you wake up to discover that all your efforts are less important than emulating some fourteen-year-old miscreant.

What you can do: First, understand that your preliminary efforts haven't been wasted. Your kid probably doesn't really want to smoke. (After all, how many smokers take a deep drag on their very first cigarette and say to themselves, "Wow! What a delightful, refreshing experience"?) He just doesn't know how to deal with peer pressure. To your kid, saying "no" to people he wants desperately to please is far worse than smoking a few cigarettes.

Second, keep in mind that not all peer pressure is bad. As your kid begins spending more time away from home, identifying more with friends, and taking up interests and activities that might earn your disapproval, it's easy to picture a United Kids Revolutionary Front whose sole purpose is to undo all your good child-rearing work. Not so. Just as there are groups of kids who encourage smoking as a form of rebellion or a means to a cool image, there are other groups who frown on smoking and believe being able to breathe is cool.

Nor does the pressure have to be external. Many kids see a group they'd like to hang out with and conform to their codes of conduct in order to gain admission or acceptance. So your kid hasn't really turned his or her back on you and entered the netherworld, much as you might feel like that's what has happened. Keep your perspective and try some of the following:

• Watch who your kid hangs out with. Is it a smoking crowd? The chances that your kid picks up a cigarette are much greater if he or she has at least one close friend who smokes. If that's the case, don't wait until you know your child has started to smoke to say something; bring up the subject first. Don't say: "I know that kid you hang out with smokes, and if you try that sort of thing around here, believe me you're dead meat." That kind of statement rarely works, and doesn't lend itself to honest and open communication between you and your child. You might want to try something like: "That Miller kid smokes, doesn't he? Do you feel like you want to smoke when you hang out with him?"

• Talk to your kid about how to deal with peer pressure. Smoking isn't the only vice your kid's friends can lead him into, and "You're grounded" isn't the only way to deal with it. Start by explaining that "peer pressure" isn't just a friend daring him or her to smoke or attempting to shame her into having that first cigarette. Peer pressure isn't always that overt, and it isn't always external. In fact, it's probably more common for a kid to light up not out of coercion but out of simple conformity—to be like everyone else in the group. Believe me, no one likes caving in to peer pressure, so give your kid   the tools he or she needs to handle it. Practice different scenarios that might arise, and talk about how your kid can refuse the pressure to light up. One of the following might help your kid out of such a situation:

  • Just say "no." OK, it's corny and old hat, but it works for some kids. Sometimes it's the only answer to give.

  • Give a good excuse for not smoking:
    "I'm not allowed to smoke."
    "I'll get kicked off the soccer team if I smoke."
    "I prefer to breathe, thank you."
    "It's a waste of money."
    "I hate the way it makes me smell."
    "It makes me sick."

- Come up with something else to do that precludes smoking. This has the added value of reminding friends that it's smoking you mind, not them.

- If friends don't recognize or respect your reasons, walk away. Who wants to hang around with people who don't respect you?

- Encourage your kid to let you know when pressure situations arise—and praise him for "doing the right thing."

- Give your kid a fact. Although it certainly might seem that "everyone" is smoking, in fact fewer than one-fifth of the country's teenagers are regular smokers.

- Continue to support, wherever possible, those activities and groups where smoking isn't an option. Sports clubs are wonderful non-smoking alternatives (but remember, they have ashtrays in bowling alleys).

- Get to know the parents of the kids your kid hangs out with. Are they smokers? Do they condone smoking? Is their home a center for teen rebellion? Or are they, too, concerned with raising non-smoking kids? Work with other parents to (a) keep informed about your kids' activities, and (b) plan smoke-free activities and events for your kids.

- Remember that you shouldn't expect teenagers to be consistently logical, articulate, or even conscious of the reasons they do things. Understand that a teenager is hardly a fully developed human with a defensible position; it will take time for your kid to become one.

- Distant as it might be, your own experiences during adolescence can help you communicate with your kid. But

GIVE YOUR CHILDREN A HEAD START TOWARD HEALTHY LUNGS: FOCUS ON SPORTS

The CDC (Center for Disease Control) revealed studies from research journals that student athletes as a sub-group have much lower incidents of smoking because:

- Sports participation establishes greater self-confidence.

- Student athletes have an additional influence against smoking from the coaching staff.

- Peer influences to smoke decrease.

- Perceived to reduce their ability and performance levels in sporting events.

- Student athletes are more attuned to the health consequences of smoking.

- Sports especially benefits girls by increasing and maintaining high self-esteem, goal-setting, and a positive body image. Girls who play sports are 92 percent less likely to be involved with drugs.

make sure they're honest experiences and memories, not cleverly crafted fictions you come up with in order to manipulate "correct behavior."

- Some kids smoke (or use drugs, get involved in risk-taking activities, or pierce every available part of their body) because they feel angry or depressed. Though they might not recognize it, those types of behavior can be a sort of cry for help. When that's the case, the problem is a difficult one and there may be no short-term solution for a parent. If your child seems overly angry or depressed, get advice from a knowledge-able health professional about where to seek help.

The Search for Independence and Adulthood

As long as smoking remains an adult habit, some kids will see tobacco as a means of feeling grown-up. For years, smoking has been one of this country's rites of passage—along with such milestones as taking a driver's test, having that first beer, and asking someone out on a date. (Admittedly, for some kids these milestones arrive rather earlier these days.) Advertisers have played to this idea for years; soldiers marching off to World War I were given cigarettes as part of their kits, thus linking the manliness of soldiering with the presence of tobacco.

What you can do:

- Explain that the only reason most adults smoke is that they began as teenagers—and that some would dearly love to quit but they can't. They, too, wanted to feel adult, so they smoked. And when they finally became adults, and didn't feel the need to smoke, they couldn't stop. That's how the trap works.

- Talk about what independence really means. Discuss how much of your kid's daily routine would be determined by cigarettes: Would your kid have to hang out with certain people only because they smoke too, and avoid certain places because smoking wasn't allowed there? Would it mean giving up parental guidance only to let an addiction for cigarettes tell her what to do?

- Discuss what being adult *really* means. What about smoking seems adult? The fact is most adults *don't* smoke. Does your child actually know any adults who feel good about their smoking or who are happy to see kids take up the habit?

- Refrain from the understandable impulse to rein in your kid's attempts to grow up. Rather, give him or her constructive opportunities to act as an adult. Encourage your kid to take on some of the healthier responsibilities and freedom that come with being adult.

- Be sure to let your kid know when he handles responsibility and shows good judgment, not just when it comes to smoking, but in all areas of life. This will help bolster his self-esteem, the best defense against peer pressure.

Part of growing up is experimenting with new behavior, new attitudes, and, often, new substances. Just as your kid might give coffee a try, he or she might want to see what smoking is about, just out of curiosity. Let your child know that this is the kind of thing you want to hear about, so you can talk about it together.

Have a little contest by challenging your kid to find one adult who will state categorically that smoking is good, and that he's glad to see kids taking up the habit. (If one is found, ascertain just how much stock this person owns in Philip Morris.) In this contest, there should be a prize when your kid loses.

The Romance of Risk and Rebellion: Too Cool to Care

Some kids turn to tobacco as a form of rebellion, just as they might wear odd clothes in order to show their distaste

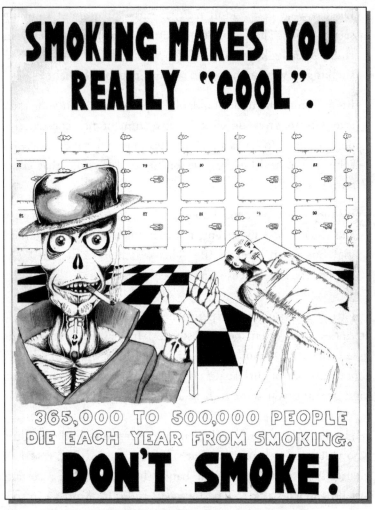

James J. Conte, Richmond Hill High School, Queens, N.Y. © 1991.

Smokefree Educational Services, Inc., NY, NY

for all things Good and Parental. And some kids light up (so they say) simply because smoking is bad for them, because it sets them apart as loners, and justifies their feelings of isolation. Many kids feel that they've been so "good" for so long, that there are so many agencies looking out for their welfare, that they've earned the right as young adults to do something that is just plain bad for them. One teen smoker, Mike, said"[Smoking] sort of changed who I hung out with at school. I was always with the good kids, and I still am, but now some of the bad kids talk to me too." Rebel smokers enjoy being defiant members of an oppressed minority, setting themselves up against "do-gooders" who play by the rules. Some take up smoking in order to prove that they're strong enough to handle it.

How many of us haven't wanted to break out of the herd and do something completely unexpected, bold, daring, or risky? How many haven't ever felt alienated from and resentful toward the whole world? Remember what life was like as a teenager, and how often you felt as though no one was going through the same pain, doubts, fears, and uncertainty as you. Remember the temptation to just give up trying to do what's right; after all, at that age it often seems that doing what's wrong is a whole lot easier.

Add to this the admiration we often feel for rule-breaking loners, and it's not hard to see why many teens take this route. Popular culture is filled with characters who succeed by going against the grain. In fact, what was once considered an innovation—the antihero—is now more commonplace than the straight-shooting good guy, who these days is more likely to be the buffoon than the hero.

Now, this is not to say that antiheroes are Bad Things and should be done away with, or that our admiration for eccentric, misunderstood loners is misplaced. It's just that our culture is loaded with rebel-type heroes who chain-smoke, so cigarettes often become part of a teenager's imitative package, a way of saying "who cares" to society.

What you can do: To the extent that you're still able to talk to your kid (it's tough getting silent rebel types to open up, unless what you're after is grunted curses), you can try a couple of things.

- Remind your kid of the difference between image and substance. How many times has he or she seen his or her smoker idols wake up in the morning hacking up phlegm?

- Talk about the fact that what your kid sees as cool rebellion is actually the result of clever marketing. Being the dupe of a tobacco company's advertising is hardly the mark of a rebel.

- Express your concern, reaffirm your opposition to smoking, and above all keep to the rules you've set. Kids often push the envelope of what is permissible, testing the limits of their independence as well as probing the seriousness of your position. A kid might simply want to provoke a reaction in his or her parents as a means of testing their commitment to her.

- Some kids take up smoking in order to push the envelope of their own limitations, to test themselves: "Hey, let's see if I can smoke and quit." If this is the case, try to involve your kid in less deadly forms of risk-taking. Hiking, swimming, and climbing are just a few activities that not only test your kid's limits but also reward fitness and good health. (And it's tough to keep your cigarettes dry in a swimming pool.)

- Mental exercises can be helpful, as well, in combating those French contributions to adolescent angst: malaise and ennui.

THE GREAT AMERICAN SMOKESCREAM

- As an outgrowth of the Great American Smokeout for adults, the American Cancer Society's Smokescream is a youth program that takes place each year the third Thursday of November: Differing in format state by state, an American Smokescream welcomes the loud, rebellious, thoughtful, concerned, angry, and even neutral youth.

- In both Minnesota and Massachusetts, youths have assembled in their state capitols to scream their message face to face with the legislatures. While adults could not get away with that, neither could a smoker.

- In 1996, the Smokescream teamed up New York and New Jersey to bring 10,000 youths together in Giant Stadium. Broadcast by one of the most popular regional radio stations, the group was entertained by rebellious, head shaved, body-pierced, anti-smoking group QKumba Zoo.

- What do you have to do to enlist your children? Call their school and tell them to call the American Cancer Society's office for your state. That's it. The school will receive a curriculum package for the students a couple of weeks before the Smokescream.

As a rule, teens see smoking not as a habit, but as an activity, something to do when they're miserable or bored. Finding ways in which to challenge themselves mentally can help fend off those moments. Encourage your kid to set and reach for goals. Saving money for a car or stereo might be using money more wisely than on cigarettes. And your contribution might be very effective in reinforcing not smoking.

Chilling Out: Smoking as Relief

One section of an old handbook on rigging concerns itself with accidents. If you witness an accident, the book reads, you should immediately summon help. Then, if the victim is conscious, the first thing you should do is *offer him a cigarette to help him calm down.*

Smoking has long been seen as a relaxing reward for the end of a stressful job, day, conversation, or duty. Many firefighters, after extinguishing fires, relax by starting a little one at the end of a cigarette. In the blockbuster movie *Independence Day*, smoking cigars was a means of celebrating a job well done, in this case, saving the human race from destruction.

But it doesn't take an invasion of aliens to make a teenager feel as though the world is about to end. Sometimes all it takes is a friend's disapproval, failure at school, or rejection by a member of the opposite sex.

Adolescence isn't just confusing; sometimes it feels downright perilous, and usually quite stressful. Your kid might feel incapable of handling the tension alone, and turn to an external source for comfort and relaxation: cigarettes. After all, cigarettes are relaxing (at least that's what the ads say), and it's some-

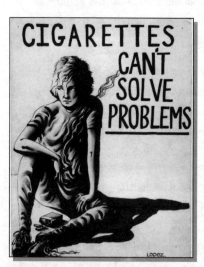

Luis Lopez, LaGuardia High School, Manhattan, N.Y. © 1991. Smokefree Educational Services, Inc., NY, NY.

thing to do when you don't know what else to do. It makes you feel as though you're in control, and gives you time to take a break and think things over.

What you can do:

•Make sure you know when your kid is feeling the heat. Keep up the regular bull sessions. Is there a specific reason your kid needs relief? Are there particular sources of stress?

•Remind your kid that you know what it feels like, not as in "You think you've got it bad; wait until you have to *yadda yadda yadda*," but as in "I know what you mean. Sometimes I get so nervous I want to scream. Here's what I do . . ."

•Set a good example by practicing good stress management yourself. (We'll assume that you don't deal with uncomfortable situations by saying, "Man, I could use a cigarette right now.")

•Make your home a place where problems are solved, not created; your kid should feel that home is a sanctuary from teenage angst. Remind your kid that there is no problem so great or so small that can't be talked about. That means, of course, that you have to listen (and I mean REALLY listen). And just like so many of the things in this book, that parental behavior needs to start well before the teen years.

WHAT IF YOUR KIDS SMOKE ANYWAY?

It can't be said too often: teenagers have a way of confounding our predictions, disappointing our expectations, surpassing our hopes, and, in general, behaving as if they had ideas of their own about how their lives are supposed to unfold. As long as tobacco is around, some number of kids—an ever-shrinking percentage, we hope—is going to end up smoking. So even if you've done everything right—set up a tobacco-free household, created positive images of non-smokers, informed your kid about the hazards of tobacco, given him or her the tools to resist aggressively manipulative marketing, helped him or her to defy peer pressure without getting ostracized, and organized your community into a haven of anti-tobacco lobbyists—there's still a chance your kid is going to end up with a cigarette dangling from his lips.

What do you do? One thought is to get extremely angry, sit your kid down, and give him a stern lecture about all you've done to safeguard him from cigarettes, and how he's a rotten little ingrate for smoking, despite all your efforts.

A better thought is to steer your kid toward quitting, not

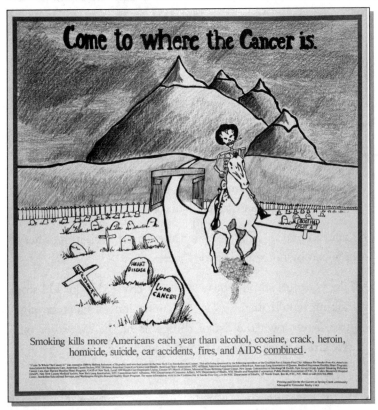

Melissa Antonow, Our Lady of Hope, Queens, N.Y. © 1991. Smokefree Educational Services, Inc., NY, NY.

by yelling or by demanding but by communicating. There are some things you can do.

- Try to find out what facet of smoking appeals to your kid, and examine it frankly.

- Don't bother reciting the long-term consequences of smoking, because it's obvious that your kid has chosen immediate gratification over future well being.

• Do remind your kid about the *immediate* downside of smoking; such as most kids don't smoke and most don't like to be around those who do; less money to spend on other pursuits; shortness of breath; bad breath and yellow teeth; smelly clothes.

• Do maintain the rules you have established regarding smoking. For example, you may be tempted to relax the rule about smoking at home, perhaps to establish a truce or to keep your kid at home more. But this just says that your anti-smoking stance was simply a posture all along.

• If your kid says, "I can quit anytime I want," ask him or her to show you by not smoking for a week.

• Make your kid an offer he or she can't refuse. If your kid stops smoking, you'll match every dollar no longer spent on cigarettes. Run down the list of things he or she can do or purchase after a week, month, summer, and year.

• Lay off.

This last suggestion is your worst-case scenario. Nothing is working; your kid smokes and that's that. Everything you try backfires on you: drives her farther away, shuts him up, makes her resent you, cements the bond with his smoking pals. With some kids, this is going to happen. The best thing you can do in this case is to be prepared for the time your kid wants to stop smoking.

• Help develop a plan with your kid. Set a quit date. Provide information and resources. Make it a joint effort.

• Reinforce the decision to quit; there may be a host of reasons your kid isn't even aware of.

•Don't pretend life will be roses as soon as he or she quits. Prepare your kid for the times he or she will be tempted to smoke again, and give him or her tools to deal with those urges.

•Establish a reward system for not smoking, such as increased allowance, greater responsibility or freedom, even simple praise.

•Stress the natural rewards that come with quitting: freedom from addiction, improved fitness, better athletic performance, better overall appearance, more money to spend on things of value.

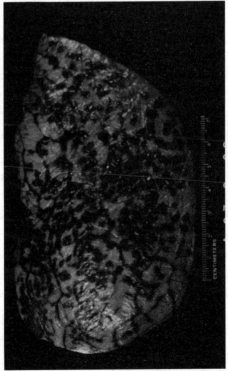

Emphysema is caused by the inhalation of toxic chemicals, such as cigarette smoke.

COMBATING MARKETING AND MYTH

Much of the anti-tobacco battle today concerns itself with the question of tobacco marketing to children. A recent study concluded that 91 percent of six-year-olds polled recognized Joe Camel as easily as they recognized Mickey Mouse—a finding that immediately catapulted Joe Camel to the top of the Parents' Hit List of Characters (knocking Barney out of the top spot).

Whatever the outcome of the debate over tobacco marketing, smoking's cultural power will be with us for some time. Even if all present means of marketing tobacco are somehow eradicated, smoking's colorful, romantic, and misleading past still presents a threat to your kids. How can you counter the long-standing American myths about smoking? How do you ensure that your kids aren't going to accept whatever marketing strategy the tobacco companies come up with next?

Explode the myth. Show your kids—and discover for yourself as well—the mechanisms behind the marketing by laying bare the reality behind the myth. This process is the difference between blind acquiescence and *critical thinking*, one of the best tools you can give your child. It will serve him or her well not only when it comes to smoking, but also with other decisions: what kind of car to buy, whom to vote for, where to live, what to accept as fact, and what to question as distortion.

Being able to explode smoking's myth and marketing is especially crucial for you and your kid because of the way tobacco insinuates itself into your kid's life. Let's take a look at how it works.

In a way, adolescence is the no-man's land between childhood and adulthood. On one side is a child wholly dependent on parents for wisdom, guidance, and sustenance. On the other side stands an adult with a life and identity of his or her own, both legally and socially responsible for making independent decisions about life. And somewhere in the middle, through a process of exploration and experimentation, we discover what it means to grow up.

Adolescence is, in many ways, the best of times and the worst of times, filled with equal parts of excitement and fear, brash confidence and painful doubt. What's right? What's wrong? What am I going to do with my life? Who am I? Suddenly, we discover that life is filled with frightening questions—and we're filled with an urgency to find the answers.

Given a choice, most of us would choose to be attractive, smart, well-liked, cool, confident, strong, and fearless. We look for ways to become those things. And even if some of those methods might seem silly later, or if some of the attitudes we adopt feel wrong, we do it because if we can't yet feel good about ourselves, at least we can *look* like we know what we're doing. We can hang out at the right places and speak

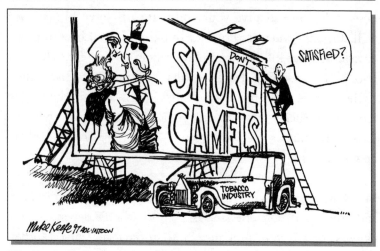

Mike Keefe/*The Denver Post*/dePiXion Studios, Inc.

the right language. We can wear the right clothes and listen to the right music with the right crowd.

And we can smoke. As a matter of fact, if you believe what tobacco advertisements tell you, smoking is the best way to achieve the "right" things. Smokers hang out at the cool places, listen to great music, have huge amounts of fun together, look great and feel confident, and share the same wonderful hobby. Even if we decide that we don't want to be part of a crowd, that life is just a big mess we have to put up with, smoking is right for us, too, because cigarettes are also the mark of the loner, the hip cynic, the rebel, and the wise.

The right clothes, the cool places, the hip attitudes—these are some of the things we try on for size as we move through adolescence. And if we eventually discover that some (or all) of them don't really fit us, they help us to get through a difficult and scary time. Once we achieve maturity, and realize that wearing the right clothes doesn't really mean a whole lot, that we really prefer listening to some other kind of music, we drop those habits and attitudes that no longer reflect who we are. And we quit smoking.

Oops. We don't quit smoking. We *can't* quit smoking. Even once we come to realize that smoking doesn't make you attractive, doesn't make you smarter, or cooler, we can't quit. Even when we realize that what smoking actually does is make us unattractive, unhealthy, and unwanted, we can't quit. Because it's too late. We're addicted to a powerful drug. We've fallen victim to one of the oldest con games in the world.

Smoking is nothing more than the old bait-and-switch: offer something desirable for sale at a great price, then deliver something that no one would buy at any price. Smoking promises anything you want. You think you're buying a great old American tradition, and what you're really getting is a deadly addiction. And the beautiful part about it is that by the time you realize you've been hoodwinked, it's too late.

If explaining all of this seems a little too abstract for your kid, you might want to compare smoking's addiction cycle with something a little closer to home—for example, clothing:

You know that baseball cap that you wear backward all the time? It's pretty cool—everyone says you look great, you hang out with a bunch of other people who wear their caps the same way. Then, one day, you graduate from high school and decide you don't want to wear your hat anymore. Maybe you don't think it's cool anymore, or maybe it's too hot to wear it. For whatever the reason, you take it off.

But five minutes later you start thinking about your hat. For some reason you feel a growing need to put on that hat. So you do. You don't like the hat, you don't want to wear it, but somehow you just feel you have to. And it goes on like that. You start carrying the hat around with you, because you can't stand not having it for long periods of time. As you get older, you begin to feel a little foolish wearing your hat all the time—but you can't stop. At work, you leave the building frequently in order to stand out on the street with your hat on. People walk by and laugh at you, shake their heads. "Another hat addict," they say.

Now imagine that you wake up one day and remember something that you've known for years, but somehow never really thought about: hats give you brain cancer.

There are many things we do as kids to make ourselves feel good (or less bad or give ourselves a good reason to feel bad), and many of them are temporary. Smoking is not one of them. It's a trap. The sign says, "Whatever you want, it's here," and you walk in. But you're not leaving, not even when you discover there's really nothing inside.

That's how smoking works. It takes advantage of the fact that you're vulnerable, that there are things you crave, and offers relief. And by the time you realize that smoking is a bogus cure for what ails you, you can't quit. You've been marketed.

It is important to understand that marketing in itself is not an evil thing nor is it solely responsible for teenage smoking. Believing that advertising is the sole source of our smoking woes may be convenient, but it's simply not true. If it were, then an across-the-board ban on all tobacco advertising (whatever you think of the appropriateness of such a gesture) would eradicate smoking, and parents would only have to worry about body piercing and loud music.

But advertising is fundamentally an opportunistic venture.

It takes advantage of popular desires and demands. Rarely is it able to create demand; usually it helps to perpetuate and reinforce demand, and to channel it toward a particular product or brand. Kids want Nike shoes not because the company created a demand for sneakers. Kids want Nike shoes because they want to be like Michael Jordan, and Michael Jordan wears Nike shoes because Nike pays him to. That's taking advantage of a kid's need to identify with heroes and role models.

Nor is marketing only effective when it comes to kids. Take, for example, the flood of psychic hotline infomercials late at night. Did these infomercials create a demand for so-called soothsayers? Hardly. Like children, adults have wishes that marketers can use to sell product. Adults call psychic hotlines not because advertisers created a demand for psychics but because adults want answers to life's questions, and businesspeople pay telephone operators to offer answers over the phone.

So marketing takes advantage of our needs and desires rather than creates them—which is why commercials are usually about a particular brand of product rather than about the product itself. For every generic "Got Milk?" ad, there are hundreds of commercials devoted not to detergents, sodas, and automobiles, but to Tide, Coke, and Saturn.

What sets smoking apart as a marketed product is not just that it's dangerous, but that it is dangerous and *addictive.* Almost everything you see advertised makes implicit (and often explicit) claims that have little to do with the actual use of the product. Once you discover that these claims are either exaggerated, completely subjective, or just plain false, you abandon the brand or the product. Every day some teenager realizes that his basketball playing is no better whether he wears a Chicago Bulls No. 23 jersey or a white T-shirt. Or you may simply no longer care about what the product offers. As you read this, somewhere some kid is looking in disgust at the last bag of Gummi Skeletons he's ever going to buy.

But almost every smoker and ex-smoker knows what follows that first moment of disgust with tobacco: another cigarette. The honeymoon might be over, but the marriage continues.

Defeating the marketing and mystique of tobacco is an essential step in raising a non-smoking kid, and involves

- understanding smoking's cultural history,

- exposing the ways in which marketing attempts to manipulate people into smoking and then supplies smokers with rationalizations for the habit,

- redefining "cool," "refreshing," "attractive," and all those other adjectives that teenagers might seek through smoking.

The first two aren't difficult, as long as you're able to communicate with your kid, and they can be fun as well. The third is rather more difficult. It will certainly take time, and there is no guarantee of success. After all, we're talking about a cultural battle. But is it so unreasonable to expect success? What we're really trying to do is depict smoking for what it truly is: unhealthy, smelly, expensive—in a word, uncool.

Understanding Tobacco's Cultural History

Kids often wonder why they're not supposed to smoke, when only a generation ago, smoking was just about the coolest, most glamorous thing you could do for half a buck. Why are there so many tobacco supporters? Why isn't tobacco illegal if it's so bad? Why does the president of the United States smoke cigars?

You should jump for joy when you hear these questions. The simple answer is: "We didn't always know smoking was bad for you." That response, however, misses a tremendous opportunity for you and your kid to discover together how smoking became an integral part of our culture. Instead of having a straight "You ask, I answer" session, the two of you can carry out your own investigation, digging up interesting facts along the way—and believe me, there aren't a lot of interesting facts that *support* smoking. Instead of passively listening to you talk about smoking, your kid can take an active role in uncovering tidbits like these:

- Marlboro, the supposed cigarette of choice for rugged, outdoorsy cowboy types, was once marketed as a woman's cigarette under the slogan "Mild as May;"

- The U.S. Armed Forces became partners with the tobacco industry every time this country went to war, handing out free cigarettes to men in uniform as standard practice. Cigarettes thus became part of a soldier's everyday life—to relieve the stress of battle and boredom and to use as currency in foreign lands. The tricky ploy of including cigarettes with food rations worked all too well, addicting those defending our country. The percentage of smoking men in the country skyrocketed. Many soldiers survived the enemy bullets and bombs, only to end their lives with the ticking bombs of tobacco-caused cancer and emphysema.

Turning the Tables on the Image-Meisters

Advertisers spend billions to get underneath your kid's skin, but you can beat them at their own game. Show your kid what advertising is all about. If you start young enough, not only will your kid be less susceptible to cigarette marketing but you might not have to change brands of cereal every other week.

FACT SHEET:
KIDS AND TOBACCO ADVERTISING

- Each year, more than 947 million packs of cigarettes are sold illegally to children under eighteen. That's 2.6 million packs a day accounting for $1.26 billion in annual sales which breaks down to $221 million worth of tobacco profits.

- Every day in the United States, 3,000 young people begin to smoke—that's more than 1 million new smokers a year.

- Ninety percent of new smokers are children and teens. These new smokers replace the smokers who die prematurely from tobacco-related diseases.

- "Old Joe," the cartoon camel used to advertise Camel cigarettes, is as familiar to six-year-old children as Micky Mouse's silhouette. A study found that ninety-one percent of six-year-olds not only recognized the Joe Camel image, but were able to correctly link him with cigarettes. This was the same recognition level measured for the Disney icon.

Dissect an advertisement

Take a look at some tobacco advertisements with your kid, and together answer the following questions:

People in the ad

• Do they look and act differently from smokers you see every day? Do they look uniformly successful and attractive? Is that

---

• The nicotine industry spends more money to promote nicotine addiction in 20 minutes than we spend in a year to prevent it.

• The 1994 surgeon general's report concluded that cigarette advertising appears to increase young people's risk of smoking.

• School-based tobacco-use prevention programs in the U.S. have had consistently positive effects. They have been particularly effective in delaying the onset of tobacco use.

• The tobacco industry doubled its advertising and promotion budget from $3.3 billion in 1988 to $6 billion in 1993. Increasingly, these marketing dollars pay for promotional activities that may have special appeal to young people, such as sponsoring rock concerts, sporting events, distributing specialty items bearing logos, and issuing coupons and premiums.

• Tobacco company spending for specialty gift items (such as T-shirts, caps, sunglasses, key chains, calendars, and sporting goods) bearing cigarette logos increased by 122 percent from $340 million in 1992 to $756 million in 1993.

an accurate picture? Look at some regular smokers. What would the ad look like if it featured these real smokers?

- Do you think the ad implies that buying the same cigarettes will make you as attractive, successful, and/or popular as the models?

- How yellow are their teeth?

- How do they smell? (Oh, you can't smell them? How fortunate.)

- Are there clouds of smoke around them, or are their cigarettes apparently burning smokelessly?

- How do you think these people would look if they weren't being paid to smoke and look happy and successful? Have you ever actually seen anyone acting this way in real life?

- Are they doing things you never see smokers doing? Why do you think so many tobacco ads feature energetic, athletic people engaged in healthy, outdoorsy activities? Think about it, how many top tennis players do you see lighting up after winning at Wimbledon?

Background and scenery

- If you see a two-page magazine ad, where is the surgeon general's warning with respect to the actual ad copy? (On different pages? How odd!)

- What does background, or scenery, have to do with cigarettes, anyway? What are the advertisers trying to convey?

Text

- What is the text saying? Are the words tobacco specific, like "makes nice, thick smoke"? Or are the words generic feel-good terms like "refreshing" and "fun"? Why aren't they tobacco specific?

•Contrast the information a cigarette ad gives you (vague pleasantries) with the kind of information other products can offer (quantifiable characteristics). For example, one particular automobile offers four-wheel drive, while another gets better mileage; one type of computer has great tech support, while another has a bigger hard drive. Even though advertisements for both cars and computers might employ the same sort of imagery and braggadocio as a cigarette ad, in the end there is actually a quantifiable way to select the product you want.

In contrast, what can cigarette advertisers say about their product? It's all bad for you.

Message

•What does the ad seem to be saying? How does it make your kid feel? One of the following messages might be appropriate:

•Smoke these and you'll be well-liked. (Notice that each message also carries its converse, e.g., "If you don't smoke these, no one will like you.")

•Smoking these keeps you really thin. ("So don't smoke, fatty.")

•Smoking these makes you look *sooo* cool. ("Non-smokers are dorks.")

•Smoking these gets you handy, cool merchandise. ("What, no Marlboro fanny pack? Loser!")

•Smoking these makes you grown-up. ("Hi, non-smoking baby.")

Now talk about whether smoking actually backs up these messages. Are smokers better liked than non-smokers? Are they better tennis players? Does smoking mean you'll never get fat?

- What would your life be like if you bought into the message every ad offers?

- Why do tobacco ads rely so heavily on images rather than on information?

Build your own ad

Once your kid gets an idea of how advertising works, see if he can come up with the following:

- An ad that is just as misleading as those you've seen. Encourage him to make the claims as outrageous as he wants, like "Smoke these and your pants will last forever!"

- An ad that reflects reality. Try to create an ad that includes known facts about cigarettes, like they're addictive; they impair your ability to breathe; they are the leading cause of cancer in this country; and they give you bad breath.

It's easy to see why cigarette advertising relies on image rather than on substance—the best truth-based ad for tobacco might be something like "Deadly . . . but *cheap!*"

Redefining Cool

If we could only find the one kid who determines what's cool and buy him or her off, redefining "cool" would be a snap.

Most of us lose our sense of cool. We reach adulthood, and can only wonder at many of the things our kids do, while taking some solace in the fact that they, too, will find themselves at a loss when their own children start acting up. When it comes to smoking, however, it's not enough to wonder why this nasty habit has maintained its coolness through the years; the stakes are too high.

So how do we go about redefining what's cool?

A first step is to recognize that cool is an attitude—and, as such, can only be changed by changing attitudes. For years we've been drumming the nasty facts about smoking into our kids' heads, only to see teenage smoking increase as it decreased in every other segment of the population. Why? Because we offered no constructive alternative to the benefits that smoking offered kids. While the tobacco industry reinforced and promoted teenage smoking through billion-dollar campaigns and state-of-the-art market research, anti-tobacco forces focused on disseminating the facts about smoking with a counter campaign based on tobacco's negative aspects. The result? A generation of well-informed kids who smoke anyway.

Keeping kids away from tobacco demands a proactive approach, one that emphasizes the positive aspects of not smoking. It's not enough to tell kids that smoking isn't cool; we have to help them realize that *not* smoking is. Only by making the concept of "cool" our own can we overcome the lure of tobacco.

But cool is a group attitude, a cultural phenomenon. To redefine it we need to act in concert with schools, communities, and nationwide organizations, and we need to employ all the tools at our disposal, including the very weapons the tobacco companies use to attract teenage smokers. We need to

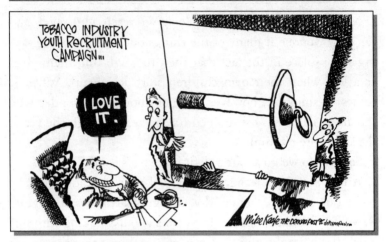

Mike Keefe/*The Denver Post*/dePIXion Studios, Inc.

involve kids in the process, make them not just participants and recruits but owners of "non-smoking cool."

Promoting non-smoking has to be an organized effort utilizing the same tools tobacco companies have used for years.

- *Media campaigns.* Well-funded private organizations can mount advertising campaigns in magazines, on television, in subways, and on billboards that promote fitness as well as counter the myths about smoking.

- *Celebrity-role model endorsements.* For every big-time star who parades around with a cigar in his mouth, there are hundreds who shudder at the very thought of lighting up. It's time to get celebrities to celebrate the fact that they don't smoke. There are, after all, far more non-smokers than smokers, and we should elicit their testimonials. By their very numbers, non-smoking role models can swamp their smoking counterparts. The opposite side of the coin is what is happening lately in movies: an increased use of tobacco to set an image. Some of this is the writer's or director's doings, often it is the result of paid "product placement" by tobacco companies or advertisers. Either way, it's wrong and filmmakers, writers, and actors need to hear from concerned parents.

- *Merchandising.* Cigarette companies don't have to be the only ones who distribute gear. Giveaways of CDs, sports equipment, T-shirts, watches, mountain bikes, and concert tickets can be used to reward non-smoking activities such as non-smoking pledge drives and competitions. Retailers can be enlisted (or pressured, if necessary) to stock the same merchandise.

- *Concerts.* Imagine a series of popular music shows with one common theme—no one smokes.

- *Press coverage.* Instead of report after report about the latest congressional hearings or recent developments in tobacco settlement talks, imagine a flood of reports about non-smoking kids' events: road rallies, concerts, sports contests, walkathons, and competitions.

- *Corporate assistance.* A nationwide program stands a good chance of pressuring corporations to choose which side of the smoking fence they're going to come down on.

Through parents' groups, non-smoking organizations, school programs, and community groups, we can start sending a different message to kids: Not smoking is the thing to do. It means energizing the silent 80 percent of teenagers who don't smoke, and getting them to applaud themselves for not smoking. Nowhere better can we apply the maxim to "think globally, act locally."

You can help redefine cool on a much smaller scale as well. For every distant celebrity who is the model of cool, there's someone in the immediate neighborhood, too, whom your kid admires:

- •an older student,

- •a local broadcasting celebrity,

- •a hometown hero—police officer, fireman, or scientist,

- •a favorite relative.

Enlist such people to add "not smoking" to their list of cool attributes when they make speeches or personal appearances in your community at local schools. You can also ask them to mention how uncool it is to smoke whenever they are chatting with kids. (Note: You should make sure that these people really don't smoke. Nothing's worse than a cool role model who gets spotted sneaking a cigarette.)

COMBATING THE COMPULSION TO SMOKE

It has often been said that in sports, "the best defense is a good offense." The same is true with respect to smoking. Rather than reacting when your kid feels the lure of tobacco, you and your child can become active agents against smoking.

School

A new saying goes: "Know your kid's school, know your kid." Naturally, you want to keep informed about what goes on when your kid is in school. And as far as smoking is concerned, there are steps you can take to make sure your kid's school sends the right message about smoking.

- Ask about educational materials and programs relating to smoking. Do you think they're sufficient? Do you have any suggestions for programs you've heard about?

- Make sure art classes no longer teach kids how to make clay ashtrays.

- Make sure the school doesn't condone smoking by students or teachers. A teacher is often the first adult role model a kid has outside the family; you don't want one of the unspoken lessons to be that smoking is OK. Insist that school, like your home, be a tobacco-free zone. Once upon a time, teacher's lounges (that mysterious haven of adult off-limits behavior) were filled with the haze of tobacco smoke. Thankfully, that's now rarely the case. Where it did exist (or still does exist), it sends a powerful message to kids who, despite their protests to the contrary, see teachers as powerful role-models.

- Ask whether teachers are well-versed in smoking prevention programs.

- Ensure that school sports are open only to non-smokers, and that none of the coaches smoke. In West Virginia, a high school football team was penalized fifteen yards because their coach's smoking on the sidelines was considered unsportsman-like conduct.

Community

The wheels of government grind slowly, and often end up turning the wrong way. Relying on federal legislation and regulation to deal with tobacco sales in your community can't be as effective as local persuasion, pressure, and action. As long as there's profit in selling tobacco, many businesses will look the other way when kids come calling. Hit these businesses where it hurts: in the wallet. Organize and participate in community programs that focus on smoking.

• Lobby to keep community events from being sponsored by tobacco companies who plaster their logos and products across the landscape. Support events with sponsors who take a non-smoking stance.

• Organize a grassroots effort to persuade convenience stores to remove tobacco advertising from their businesses and remove "loosies" (cigarettes sold individually).

• Lead or join a movement to boycott businesses that carry cigarette vending machines.

• Set up a sting operation with local law enforcement using neighborhood kids. The CDC's Youth Risk Behavior Study shows that three out of four high school students were not asked to show proof of age when buying cigarettes. See how easy it is for them to purchase cigarettes in your area, and then bust the retailers. (This sort of thing goes over big with local newspapers and television stations.)

• Hook up with a national organization that sponsors community events, like the American Cancer Society or Stop Teenage Addiction to Tobacco (STAT). Such groups have a wealth of activities, booklets, T-shirts, posters, newsletters, contests, and conferences to offer.

• Sponsor a contest for the best "Reality-Based Cigarette Campaign," with fitness-related prizes.

• Organize or take part in a letter-writing campaign to local newspapers, lawmakers, and business owners.

Online

There's a wealth of non-smoking information and activities to be found on the World Wide Web. If you have a computer with Internet access, you and your kid can browse the non-smoking resources online such as taking part in Web projects, joining chat groups, reading up on the latest info, and learning what other kids are doing instead of smoking. "Surfing the net" with your kid not only gives him the opportunity to teach you how to use the computer, but also gives you both the chance to do the following:

- contact non-smoking kids outside of your immediate area (Since a common teenage misconception is that "everyone is doing it," exposure to countless kids around the world who aren't doing it can open your kid's eyes),

- learn how other organizations, school groups, and community concerns are dealing with the question of kids' smoking,

- get in touch with parents' groups and learn from their successes and failures.
  Here are just a few selected sites to get you started:

- **KidsHealth** (Nemours Foundation) (http://www.kidshealth.org);

- **Action on Smoking and Health** (ASH) (http://ash.org);

- **American Cancer Society** (http://www.cancer.org);

- **Washington DOC** (Doctors Ought to Care) (http://kickbutt.org);

- **Campaign for Tobacco-Free Kids**
  (http://www.tobaccofreekids.org);

- The Massachusetts Tobacco Education Clearinghouse (http://www.quitnet.org);

- The Tobacco BBS (http://www.tobacco.org).

You should also know that there are countless Web sites devoted to smokers' rights, such as smoking as a Great Thing, smoking as a fetish, smoking as a Multinational Conspiracy to Orchestrate the Vegan Animal Rights Activist Takeover of the World. There are even sites applauding teen smoking, some run by teenagers themselves. Rather than avoid such sites and risk being seen as an Evil Parental Censor of Truth when your kid finds them, stop by some of these sites with your kid and discuss what they're all about.

A QUIZ FOR YOU AND YOUR KIDS

Here's a little quiz to test you and your kid's knowledge of smoking. Take it together. Talk about what the answers mean. And for Pete's sake, keep it light. Nothing turns a kid off more than earnestness. The goal here is to pass along information by communicating, not by lecturing.

1. A few drops of nicotine on your tongue will

   a. kill you

   b. relax you

   c. make your tongue numb

   d. freshen your breath

Answer: **a.** Nicotine is an oily, colorless liquid used in many insecticides, and there is enough of it in a typical cigar to kill you twice over. The good news is that absorbing nicotine through inhaled smoke is vastly inefficient, so smokers don't

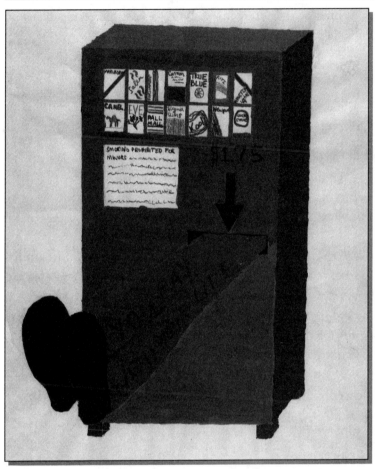

Culleen Duffy, Nightingale-Bamford School, Manhattan, N.Y. © 1991.

keel over immediately. Instead, they absorb just enough of it to experience that soothing nicotine "high." The bad news is that the subsequent addiction to nicotine keeps millions of people smoking until they do finally keel over—from lung cancer, heart disease, emphysema, or a host of other smoking-related ailments.

2. Which of the following is NOT a possible result of using smokeless tobacco?

a. oral cancer

b. gum inflammation

c. tooth decay

d. receding gums

e. tooth loss

f. whiter teeth

Answer: **f.** Smokeless tobacco, or chewing tobacco, is simply another way of delivering nicotine to the body—when that lovely brown tobacco juice is absorbed through the lining of the mouth. Users of smokeless tobacco trade the risk of lung cancer for the risk of mouth cancer.

3. Which of the following chemicals is present in cigarette tobacco?

a. cyanide

b. benzene

c. formaldehyde

d. methanol (wood alcohol)

e. acetylene

f. ammonia

g. all of the above

Answer: **g.** All these chemicals are present in cigarette tobacco and dozens more. Do you really want to deposit a veritable toxic waste dump into your lungs?

4. A survey of high school students who were daily smokers revealed that only 5 percent intended to still be smoking in 5 years. What percentage was still smoking 5 years later?

   a. 5 percent

   b. 10 percent

   c. 50 percent

   d. 75 percent

Answer: **d.** You can guess why: Smoking isn't just a habit but an addiction. The reasons people keep smoking are far removed from the reasons they took up smoking:

   "I though I'd just try it . . . but I just can't seem to quit."
   "Everyone else was doing it. Now no one can stop."
   "It made me feel like an adult, now I just feel old."
   "I wanted to lose weight . . . and ended up losing a lung."

5. On the average, someone who smokes a pack a day loses how many years of life?

   a. three

   b. five

   c. seven

   d. twenty-five

Answer: c. If only it were twenty-five years, fewer people would smoke, don't you think? Maybe they should think about making cigarettes more lethal. How close does probable disease, disability, and death have to be to seem real?

6. Teenage smokers do something twice as much as non-smoking teenagers. What is it?

    a. Get dates.

    b. Graduate from high school.

    c. Earn varsity letters in sports.

    d. Produce phlegm.

Answer: d. And believe me, excessive phlegm doesn't rate very high on anyone's Dream Date list. Nor is it particularly helpful academically. Nor is it a sign of a true sports champion.

7. Which of the following statements are false?

    a. only heavy smokers die

    b. stopping smoking after many years has little effect

    c. smoking only kills people in old age

    d. there are comparable causes of cancer

Answer: They're all false. Let's take them one at a time.

    a. *Only heavy smokers die*: "Heavy" is a relative term. You don't have to smoke two packs a day to suffer or even die from a smoking-related illness.

b. *Stopping smoking after many years has few benefits*: In fact, your body begins undoing the damage caused by smoking each time you don't light a cigarette (a smoker's early morning cough is the result of eight hours' recovery by the lungs). Quitting at any stage improves your odds of avoiding smoking-related problems, such as acute bronchitis or pneumonia. That says nothing of the immediate benefits of not smoking: fewer cigarette burns in clothing and on furniture, a home and body that feel fresh, more money to spend on things that don't kill you.

c. *Smoking only kills people in old age*: How old is old? Steve McQueen died at fifty, Nat King Cole at forty-five. Although John Wayne died at seventy-two, he probably would have liked to have a few more years. People have varying reactions to cigarettes, and some smokers exacerbate problems that, without smoking, might not prove fatal.

This doesn't count the number of people who fall asleep with cigarettes in their hands and burn to death, or those who drop a cigarette on themselves while driving and swerve into trees trying to retrieve it.

Besides, smoking doesn't just kill you. First, it poisons your life, and *then*, it kills you.

d. *There are comparable causes of cancer*: Nice try. Lung cancer kills more people than any other cancer, and almost 90 percent of lung cancer is attributed to smoking.

8. True or false? Tobacco is responsible for the following effects on the body: rapid heart beat and higher pulse rates; shortness of breath and reduced circulation; increased coughing; greater susceptibility to colds, flu, and pneumonia

a. True (but look at the upside: Cancer)

b. False (more propaganda generated by those anti-tobacco forces who have normal pulses, higher lung capacity, and greater resistance to colds)

9. How many tries does it take the average adult to finally quit smoking?

a. 2

b. 3

c. 4

d. 5

e. Does dying count?

Answer: **d.**

10. For the movie *Superman II*, the producers decided that intrepid *Daily Planet* reporter Lois Lane should smoke Marlboro cigarettes. Why?

a. the actress who played Lois Lane was a smoker, and couldn't get through any of her scenes without lighting up

b. it was an easy way to show that Lois was a strong, cool, confident, independent, attractive, capable woman

c. it was an easy way to show that Lois Lane was a weak, addicted, fearful, smelly, wrinkled woman

d. the makers of Marlboros gave a heap of money to the producers

Answer: **d**. I guess the producers had too much backbone to have Superman smoke Marlboros. But if you think about it, Superman would have been a better choice. He's invulnerable, so smoking couldn't harm him. It's only we earthlings, born under a yellow sun, who end up dying of emphysema.

11. What is the most common therapeutic use for nicotine?

a. antidepressant

b. local anesthetic

c. antispasmodic

d. vitamin B supplement

e. Nice try, there isn't one

Answer: **e**. How did you guess? Nicotine has no known therapeutic use. But as we saw in the first question, it's a real good poison!

12. Clove cigarettes contain

a. no tobacco, no tar, no nicotine, no flavor

b. a mentholating agent that filters out tar

c. more tar and nicotine than regular cigarettes

d. tiny alien critters

e. aromatherapeutic herbs

Answer: **c**. If only it *were* tiny alien critters; they're probably better for you than tar. But trust me, if tiny alien critters were combined in a cigarette with nicotine, you'd see a lot of people standing outside office buildings with "E.T." cigarettes.

13. Smoking was introduced to this country by

  a. Christopher Columbus

  b. Sir Walter Raleigh

  c. Lady Virginia Slim

  d. Leif Eriksson

  e. Leaf Tobaccoson

  f. everyone's favorite: none of the above

Answer (all together now): **f.** The natives of San Salvador were smoking tobacco when Columbus arrived. Tobacco leaves were among the first gifts given to Columbus's men, who, not understanding what to do with them, tossed them. But they soon learned that the leaves were for smoking.

14. Inhaled nicotine reaches the brain in approximately how many seconds?

  a. one to three seconds

  b. three to five seconds

  c. ten to nineteen seconds

  d. thirty to forty-five seconds

  e. sixty seconds

Answer: **c.** If only common sense could be as quickly inhaled.

15. What fraction of smokers have a cigarette within 10 minutes of waking up in the morning?

    a. one-tenth

    b. one-third

    c. one-half

    d. two-thirds

    e. nine-tenths

Answer: **b.** One-third of all smokers can't wait ten minutes before having a cigarette in the morning.

16. What fraction of smokers have a cigarette within thirty minutes of waking up in the morning?

    a. one-tenth

    b. one-third

    c. one-half

    d. two-thirds

    e. nine-tenths

Answer: **d.** Two-thirds of all smokers manage to hold out for thirty minutes. Now *that's* willpower! Imagine how these people feel in a restaurant, theater, classroom, or airplane after forty-five minutes.

17. Tobacco is considered a "gateway" substance. This means that tobacco users

   a. are more likely to be found standing outside buildings

   b. are more likely to get into chic night spots

   c. are more likely to use drugs like alcohol, marijuana, cocaine, and heroin

   d. are more likely to surf the Internet

Answer: **c.**

18. Which kills more people in the United States?

   a. automobile accidents

   b. tobacco

   c. gunfire

   d. AIDS

Answer: **b**, of course. In fact, tobacco-related deaths account for more people dying than the other three combined.

19. Cigar smokers are three times as likely to _____ as non-smokers

   a. own BMWs

   b. marry movie stars

   c. end up with mouth cancer

   d. win a Nobel Prize

Answer: **c.** Cigars are of no use in achieving the other three choices. BMWs cost money, so putting those cigar bucks into an interest-bearing account will do more for you in that respect. Movie stars, as a rule, only smoke when they're paid to, so you're not likely to attract one on the basis of that foul cigar. As for winning a Nobel Prize? You need smarts to do that, not tobacco.

KIDSHEALTH.ORG SMOKING POLL RESULTS

Total number of smokers polled (age 18 or younger): 25

Total number of non-smokers polled: 433

Average age of smokers: 15

Average age of non-smokers: 11

The sale of cigarettes by people younger than 18 should be illegal.

Smokers:	52% Agree	48% Disagree
Non-smokers:	92% Agree	8% Disagree

Cigarette vending machines and free samples of cigarettes should be prohibited.

Smokers:	24% Agree	76% Disagree
Non-smokers:	89% Agree	11% Disagree

Outdoor tobacco ads should be banned within 1,000 feet of schools and playgrounds.

Smokers:	36% Agree	64% Disagree
Non-smokers:	88% Agree	12% Disagree

Tobacco promotional items, such as baseball caps, t-shirts, and backpacks with cigarette logos on them should be banned.

Smokers:	20% Agree	80% Disagree
Non-smokers:	70% Agree	30% Disagree

Tobacco manufacturers should be required to sponsor a national tobacco-free education program.

Smokers:	36% Agree	64% Disagree
Non-smokers:	79% Agree	21% Disagree

Tobacco brand sponsorship of sporting and cultural events should be prohibited.

Smokers:	12% Agree	88% Disagree
Non-smokers:	65% Agree	35% Disagree

Do your parents smoke?

Smokers:	56% Yes	44% No
Non-smokers:	26% Yes	74% No

Do your grandparents smoke?

Smokers:	44% Yes	56% No
Non-smokers:	30% Yes	60% No

Do your siblings smoke?

Smokers: 44% Yes   56% No
Non-smokers: 7% Yes   93% No

Smoking is

a) very harmful to your health.
   Smokers: 25%
   Non-smokers: 92%

b) is a little harmful to your health.
   Smokers: 26%
   Non-smokers: 3%

c) doesn't affect your health
   Smokers: 24%
   Non-smokers: 0%

Smokers: I smoke because. . . (more than one selection could be chosen)

It tastes good: 64%	I just like it: 76%
It relaxes me: 72%	I don't know why: 20%
My friends smoke: 40%	I was told not to: 40%
I'm addicted: 64%	It keeps my weight down: 24%
It's cool: 20%	My parents smoke: 36%

Non-smokers: I don't smoke because. . .

It tastes bad: 48%	It's not cool: 71%
It makes me feel sick: 46%	I was told not to: 63%
I don't want to be addicted: 77%	My parents don't smoke: 57%
It's bad for my health: 89%	It's too expensive: 37%
It causes cancer: 88%	Smoking stains my teeth brown: 63%
It causes wrinkles: 50%	Smoking fills my lungs with tar: 77%
My friends don't smoke: 49%	I don't know why not: 8%

A FEW RESPONSES TO KIDS' QUESTIONS ABOUT SMOKING

Rather than responding to your kids' curiosity about smoking with the ever-handy "Because I said so," try some of the answers below.

Q. You smoke, why can't I?

A. You *really* don't want to have to answer this question. What can you say: I'm stupid? I'm a hypocrite? I'm an addict? At worst, you want the question to be "You *smoked*; why can't I?" Even that one is hard to answer, but at least you can come up with a defensible position: explain why you started ("No one asked me to, but everyone I hung out with was smoking, so I just joined in"); why you wanted to stop ("I wanted to be able to take a deep breath, to taste things again, to run my own life"); how hard it was to stop ("It took me three tries, and it was pretty awful for a while"); and what your life is like now ("I can run again; I don't carry the smell of cigarettes wherever I go; I figure I've saved a few thousand bucks since I stopped smoking").

Q. Uncle Winston has been smoking for twenty years, and there's nothing wrong with him. So what's the big deal?

A. For one thing, Uncle Winston might be one of the few very lucky smokers who manage to die of something other than a smoking-related disease. The odds, however, are against him. In fact, according to the American Lung Association one of every three deaths among older men who smoke more than a pack of cigarettes a day is related to smoking. So your Uncle Winston is still taking a one in three chance that he'll die from smoking.

But the fact that Uncle Winston is alive isn't the only thing to consider. You have to look at how he lives his life. In fact, he doesn't. Cigarettes run his life. His addiction to nicotine runs his life. He may look cool smoking and may not show any signs of impending doom, but watch what happens if you stick Uncle Winston in a movie theater for three hours. He sits there, watching the movie, and after a while his addiction starts talking to him. "Don't you wish you could smoke right now?" it says. "Hey, that guy in the movie is smoking. Don't you want a cigarette, too?" Uncle Winston tries to keep his mind on the movie, but part of his brain is calculating how long before he can smoke, how relieved he's going to feel when he steps outside and lights one up. Then his addiction starts talking again: "This movie isn't that good, anyway. You won't miss anything if you step outside to have a smoke. Go ahead. Do it."

Finally, Uncle Winston can't take it anymore. He goes outside and has a cigarette. As the nicotine enters his bloodstream, he resolves not to go to the movies as much anymore. It will be better to watch them on video at home, where he can chain-smoke and watch at the same time.

Uncle Winston's life is full of such moments. He no longer makes choices based on his wants; he makes them based on his need for nicotine. He's a prisoner.

And how often does Uncle Winston feel like going outside and tossing the football around? How long does he last before he either has to quit, or sit down and have a smoke? If you could choose someone who had to run and get help in an emergency, would you pick Uncle Winston—or someone who could breathe?

Still think there's "nothing wrong" with Uncle Winston?

Q. They can't even say what part of smoking is the cause of lung cancer. Doesn't that mean it might not be true?

A. It's true that the exact component that is responsible for lung cancer hasn't been identified. Neither has the exact cause of the TWA crash, but that doesn't mean that no one died.

Q. That TV commercial says if you just use the patch you can quit smoking. Why can't I just do that when I feel like quitting?

A. The patch, like other drug therapies, addresses only one part of smoking addiction: nicotine dependency. But smoking also has a psychological component that, in many ways, is even harder to overcome. By the time you decide to quit, tobacco will have become such an integral part of your everyday life that you'll find it hard to imagine life without it. Smokers, often finding themselves wanting desperately to break free of the habit, ask themselves anguished questions like: *How can I have my cup of morning coffee without a smoke?*

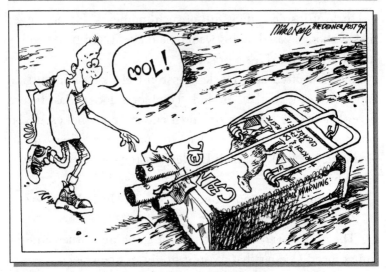

Mike Keefe/ *The Denver Post*/ dePIXion Studios, Inc.

What am I going to do when I want to relax? What can I do with my hands? What am I going to do when I'm bored, or unhappy? What am I going to do when my smoking friends light up? What am I going to do to celebrate? What am I going to do when I'm waiting?

Nicotine replacement therapies can wean you from nicotine, but they can't fill in the gaping hole left in your daily life when you stop smoking.

Q. Hey, at least I'm not drinking and driving, right?

A. Drinking and driving is an irresponsible act that often results in grave or fatal harm immediately. Smoking is an irresponsible act that usually results in serious or fatal harm, it just takes a bit longer.

Q. If smoking were a real killer, they'd outlaw it completely, right?

A. It's certainly true that cigarettes are a commodity that, if used correctly, will kill you. But tobacco was in use in this country long before its effects on health were known. Even then, it was a while before its effects on health were *proved*. Can you imagine if cigarettes had never existed and were recently created that they would be allowed on the market? "What's this? You want to market a highly addictive product which will enable people to inhale smoke fumes containing dozens of poisonous and cancer-causing compounds which will eventually lead to heart disease and other medical problems? We don't think so!"

Q. It's OK, because I smoke low-tar cigarettes.

A. Nice try. If you switch from regular cigarettes to low-tar ones, you probably smoke more of them to make up for the fact that less nicotine is getting into your system. Everyone has a different tolerance for nicotine. People who smoke will quickly discover the number of cigarettes they have to smoke in order to reach that level. When they switch to low tar, thinking that they can offset some of the hazards of smoking, most people smoke enough of them to reach that same level of nicotine tolerance, which means smoking more cigarettes, and inhaling much more deeply. They end up with the same amount of tar and nicotine in their system as before. And recent studies indicate that by inhaling more deeply, you drive those little tar particles even farther into your lungs, which results in a whole *new* ailment.

Q. I can smoke as long as I don't inhale.

A. In that case, why don't you forget about lighting them as well? And if you're going to go that far, why waste the money?

Aside from that, remember that smoke is never a Good Thing. Nicotine and chemicals from smoke are still absorbed through the inside of the mouth and throat, which leads to increased chances for cancer of the mouth, lips, and oropharynx. Smoke does damage. Even smokers who think they don't inhale, like pipe and cigar smokers, increase their chances of getting lung cancer by incidental inhalation.

Q. But air pollution could be just as bad for me as smoking, right?

A. Two things come to mind: you don't have to go out and buy air pollution; it's free. And you don't see a lot of people running around with their lips to exhaust pipes because they have a craving for carbon monoxide, do you?

Q. By the time I get cancer they'll have come up with a cure, right?

A. Betting your life on that isn't such a good idea. Besides, which do you think people are going to want to give their money to: an organization that fights cancer which strikes people by chance or an organization that fights cancer which you decided you didn't mind getting? Trust me, you're not going to win the sympathy vote.

Q. There are no warnings on cigar packs, so they must be OK.

A. Wrong, they are actually richer in nocious combustion products. A standard, half-ounce cigar can generate seven times as much tar as a cigarette, eleven times as much carbon monoxide, and four times as much nicotine. When U.S. Congress passed the law mandating warnings on cigarettes, they overlooked cigars—and tobacco companies weren't going to warn anyone about the hazards of smoking cigars unless they had to. After all, what they're interested in is profits, not truth. Look for this oversight to be remedied soon.

Q. I'll quit smoking when it starts hurting me.

A. That would be now. There are plenty of short-term effects of smoking: hoarseness, bad breath, decreased athletic performance, greater susceptibility to colds, stained teeth, and shortness of breath. Tell you what: race me to the end of the street. Take a few really deep breaths. It's hurting you already.

Q. I wouldn't feel the effects of quiting for years.

A. Not true. In as fast as twenty seconds after your last cigarette, the blood pressure and pulse rate drop to normal. In twenty-four hours the chance of a heart attack decreases and in forty-eight hours the nerve endings start regrowing. Imagine how you'll feel in a year!

THE HISTORY OF TOBACCO IN AMERICAN CULTURE

This is by no means a complete timeline of the history of tobacco, just some of the high, low, somewhat interesting, and downright maddening points. You and your kid should feel free to investigate on your own, and discover how nicotine got its name, how long the Smokers' Airline lasted, and what General Pershing had to say about cigarettes.

1492: Among the token gifts Columbus and his men receive from the natives of San Salvador are tobacco leaves. They have no idea that they are supposed to stick the leaves inside a pipe, set them on fire, and inhale the smoke. But they soon learn, and bring some tobacco leaves back to Europe with them. This could explain why Europe doesn't celebrate Columbus Day.

1604: England's King James I expresses his contempt for smoking in *A Counterblaste to Tobacco*: "Smoking is a custom loathsome to the eye, hateful to the nose, harmful to the brain, dangerous to the lungs, and in the black, stinking fume thereof nearest resembling the horrible Stygian smoke of the pit that is bottomless."

Loathsome it might be, but it becomes tremendously profitable for his government by way of taxation.

1609: John Rolfe sails to America from England. He settles in Virginia and begins growing tobacco, which becomes the foundation for the colony's economy.

1776: Tobacco helps finance the Revolution by serving as collateral for loans from France. And why not? By then Europe was hooked.

1861–1865: Yankee soldiers marching through the South discover the region's "bright" tobacco—a milder, sweeter, domestic tobacco—and bring it back North with them. Bright tobacco becomes immensely popular, and demand for it fuels the economic rebuilding of the South.

1875: R. J. Reynolds founds the R. J. Reynolds Tobacco Company, which markets chewing tobacco under such names as Golden Rain, Yellow Rose, and Purity. (Odd names for something that requires having a spittoon handy.)

1881: James Bonsack secures a patent for his cigarette manufacturing machine, which turns out more than 200 cigarettes a minute (as opposed to a hand roller's rate of 4 or 5 per minute). This innovation makes cigarettes both cheaper and more widely distributed.

1896: The first advertisement appears on a matchbook, which quickly becomes a "hot" item.

1899: Sunday school teacher Lucy Page Gaston, who coined the term "cigarette face" to describe one of the unpleasant effects of smoking, founds the Anti-Cigarette League of Chicago. In two years' time the league goes national, with Gaston spearheading a drive to eradicate cigarette smoking in the United States. The league lobbies for legislation to ban the sale and use of cigarettes, and pressures private firms to prohibit smoking by their employees. The league's sporadic successes during that time are overshadowed by a huge increase in cigarette sales.

In 1920, Gaston seeks the Republican presidential nomination, making repeated reference to candidate (and smoker) Warren Harding's "cigarette face." She is never considered a serious candidate, and dies four years later—of throat cancer.

1902: Philip Morris sets up shop in New York.

1909: Future baseball Hall of Famer Honus Wagner insists that his card, featured in Sweet Caporal cigarette packs, be taken out of circulation. Although a tobacco chewer, Wagner does not want his name associated with tobacco products.

The resulting shortage makes his card the most valuable in history; in 1996 a mint condition Wagner card will sell for almost $650,000.

1912: In a monograph, Dr. I. Adler is the first to strongly suggest that lung cancer is related to smoking.

1913: R. J. Reynolds introduces Camel cigarettes in a nation-wide advertising campaign.

1917–1918: During World War I, cigarettes find a place in the rations of American soldiers. General Pershing rates tobacco as highly as bullets in the war effort, and cigarettes are linked with courage, patriotism, and manhood.

1924: Philip Morris introduces Marlboro, a women's cigarette that is "Mild as May."

1928: The American Tobacco Company targets women with a new promotion for Lucky Strikes; "Reach for a Lucky Instead of a Sweet" advises women who are concerned about their weight to smoke rather than eat.

1932: George G. Blaisdell invents the Zippo lighter.

1933: Kool, a menthol cigarette, is introduced. The only other menthol cigarette on the market is named Spuds. Kool quickly becomes the top-selling menthol cigarette.

1941–1945: World War II brings on another boom in smoking as cigarettes are given to soldiers as part of their kits. Advertising on the home front never fails to remind consumers that cigarettes and heroism go hand in hand.

1942: *Now, Voyager*, starring Bette Davis and Paul Henreid, is released. The film is a milestone in the annals of smoking "cool." Henreid places two cigarettes in his mouth, lights them, then hands one to Davis. Men imitate, women swoon. If only Davis had said, "No, thanks," smoking might have looked silly instead of suave, and Davis might not have had so many strokes later in life.

1947: Singer Tex Williams has a hit with the song "Smoke! Smoke! Smoke! (That Cigarette)," which has the nerve to suggest that you can "smoke yourself to death." Williams will make the point more emphatically when he dies of lung cancer in 1985.

1950: Dancing packs of Lucky Strike cigarettes tap their way into American homes as the sponsors of *Your Hit Parade*.

1952: Kent cigarettes are introduced. They feature a special "micronite" filter that assures healthy smoking. The main ingredient in the filter? Asbestos.

1952: *Reader's Digest* magazine publishes, "Cancer by the Carton." The article sparks a boom in the popular press, and the American public is inundated by reports of a link between cigarette smoking and lung cancer. For the first time in more than two decades, cigarette sales decline.

1953: The journal *Cancer Research* prints a report by Ernst Wynder and Evarts Graham describing experiments in which cigarette tars painted onto the backs of mice resulted in cancerous tumors.

1954: When Philip Morris introduces the Marlboro Cowboy, its former slogan, "Mild as May," seems somewhat inappropriate. "Delivers the Goods on Flavor" is the new motto.

1954: Leaders of the tobacco industry retain public relations firm Hill and Knowlton to deal with mounting public awareness about the hazards of smoking. The Tobacco Institute Research Committee is formed, and runs a nationwide advertisement titled, "A Frank Statement to Tobacco Smokers." Here are a few excerpts from this frank statement:

We accept an interest in people's health as a basic responsibility, paramount to every other consideration in our business. . . .We believe the products we make are not injurious to health. . . .We always have and always will cooperate closely with those whose task it is to safeguard the public health.

We are pledging aid and assistance to the research effort into all phases of tobacco use and health. This joint financial aid will of course be in addition to what is already being contributed by individual companies. . . .For this purpose we are establishing a joint industry group consisting initially of the undersigned. This group will be known as "The Tobacco Institute Research Committee."

This statement is being issued because we believe the people are entitled to know where we stand on this matter and what we intend to do about it.

1955: Edward R. Murrow, chain-smoking CBS newsman, hosts "See It Now," which airs an episode examining the hazards of cigarette smoking. Murrow refrains from smoking on this particular program, but continues the habit. Ten years later he dies from lung cancer.

1964: "Smoking and Health: Report of the Advisory Committee to the Surgeon General" concludes that cigarette smoking is a cause of lung cancer in men—and a suspected cause in women.

1965: Congress passes the Federal Cigarette Labeling and Advertising Act, which mandates the placement of official surgeon general's warnings on cigarette packs. These warnings read, "Caution: Cigarette Smoking May Be Hazardous to Your Health." Dedicated smokers enjoy the use of the words "May Be," and tell themselves that it won't happen to them.

1966: John F. Banzhaf III petitions the Federal Communications Commission (FCC) to apply the Fairness Doctrine to cigarette commercials, and asks the commission to mandate equal time for anti-cigarette "commercials."

1967: The FCC rules that the Fairness Doctrine does indeed apply to cigarette advertising. Hence, stations that broadcast cigarette commercials must provide free air time to anti-smoking messages.

1967: A report of the surgeon general concludes that smoking is the principal cause of lung cancer. In half a century, the disease has gone from a medical curiosity to a common killer.

1967: Actor William Talman, a perennial loser as prosecutor Hamilton Burger to television's Perry Mason, appears in a commercial. He introduces his wife and six children, and goes on to say:

> You know, I didn't really mind losing those courtroom battles. But I'm in a battle right now I don't want to lose at all.

Because if I lose it, it means losing my wife and those kids you just met. I've got lung cancer. So take some advice about smoking and losing, from someone who's been doing both for years: If you don't smoke, don't start. If you do smoke, quit. Don't be a loser.

By the time the commercial airs, Talman is dead.

1968: Virginia Slims cigarettes are introduced, targeting the female market. Advertisements compare traditional women's roles with the freedom, independence, and confidence of their modern counterparts, who celebrate their independence with cigarettes. One of their most memorable slogans is "You've Come a Long Way, Baby." Feminists wonder which is worse: trying to get women to smoke or calling them "baby."

1968: At last, a "safe" cigarette, Bravo, a nontobacco cigarette made with lettuce, makes its debut. "Boo, Hiss" might have been a better name; the cigarette is a huge flop.

1969: The FCC issues a Notice of Proposed Rulemaking to ban cigarette ads on television and radio.

1970: The surgeon general's warning gets tougher with "Warning: The Surgeon General Has Determined that Cigarette Smoking Is Dangerous to Your Health."

1971: Cigarette ads disappear from television and radio. As a result, all the powerful anti-smoking public service messages disappear as well. Product placement in TV shows and motion pictures, however, continues.

1972: Marlboro becomes the best-selling cigarette in the world.

1973: The Civil Aeronautics Board mandates the establishment of non-smoking sections on all commercial airline flights.

1974: The city of Monticello, Minnesota, mimics the 1971 film *Cold Turkey*, in which an entire town goes thirty days without cigarettes to win a huge prize. Monticello stages a one-day smokeout, which in three years becomes a nationwide annual event. The prize, in this case, is good health.

1975: The U.S. Armed Forces stop handing out cigarettes to soldiers, sailors, and pilots.

1983: Arthur Godfrey dies of lung cancer. The hugely popular radio and TV personality had once signed off his Chesterfield-sponsored program with the words: "This is Arthur 'Buy-'em-by-the-carton' Godfrey."

1984: The Comprehensive Smoking Education Act expands the number of health warnings on cigarette packs and in advertisements. Cigarette manufacturers must rotate the following warnings every three months:

Surgeon General's Warning: Smoking Causes Lung Cancer, Heart Disease, Emphysema, and May Complicate Pregnancy;

Surgeon General's Warning: Quitting Smoking Now Greatly Reduces Serious Risks to Your Health;

Surgeon General's Warning: Smoking by Pregnant Women May Result in Fetal Injury, Premature Birth, and Low Birth Weight;

Surgeon General's Warning: Cigarette Smoke Contains Carbon Monoxide.

1984: Nicotine gum is introduced as a prescription cessation method.

1985: Lung cancer overtakes breast cancer as the No. 1 killer of women.

1985: Actor Yul Brynner dies of lung cancer. A videotape of him is released with the following introduction: "Ladies and gentlemen, the late Yul Brynner." The actor says, "Now that I am gone, I tell you: don't smoke. Whatever you do, just don't smoke."

1986: Patrick Reynolds, grandson of tobacco company magnate R. J. Reynolds, joins the anti-tobacco movement. In 1989 he will found the not-for-profit Foundation for a Smoke-free America.

1988: The surgeon general releases the report "Health Consequences of Smoking: Nicotine Addiction" which concludes that "cigarettes and other forms of tobacco are addicting and that actions of nicotine provide the pharmacologic basic of tobacco addiction."

1990: Smoking is banned on all scheduled domestic flights of six hours or less.

1992: The transdermal nicotine patch makes its appearance. It is available only in prescription form, as opposed to that other nicotine delivery system—cigarettes.

1992: "Marlboro Man" Wayne McLaren, fifty-one, dies of lung cancer.

1994: Seven tobacco company executives testify before the U.S. Congress that they do not believe smoking is addictive. Seeing a photograph of the executives being sworn in, many people don't know whether to laugh or cry about their obvious perjury.

1994: Mississippi files suit against the tobacco industry to recoup millions of dollars in smokers' Medicaid bills. Other states soon follow Mississippi's lead.

1994: FDA Commissioner Kessler testifies that cigarettes may qualify as drug delivery systems. Such a classification would bring tobacco under the jurisdiction of the FDA.

1995: The Food and Drug Administration finally declares nicotine a drug.

1996: The Food and Drug Administration approves the Nicotrol transdermal patch and nicotine gum for nonprescription sale.

1997: As part of a settlement of state lawsuits over Medicaid expenses, the Liggett Group admits that smoking is addictive. It is the first tobacco company to do so.

CESSATION METHODS

Whether you need to stop smoking for your own sake and the sake of your children or you need to provide your kid with the tools to stop smoking, you're going to need information on cessation. Don't wait until you hear, "When I decide to stop, I'll just get the patch," to read up on the subject. The booming cessation industry is a double-edged sword: Although there are now many well-publicized ways to quit smoking, the commercials and publicity might lead your kid to think that quitting is a simple, easy process.

Many cessation products and methods are, for the most part, businesses. Noble as their cause might be, their bottom line is . . . well, the bottom line. Their advertisements are upbeat, positive claims that their particular method is the easiest, most effective means of giving up tobacco. Makers of the patch and the nicotine gum are certainly not going to broadcast their failures or emphasize the difficulty in quitting. If they did, who would believe they could quit smoking? And who would buy their products?

The truth is that quitting is not as simple as getting a patch, chewing nicotine gum, or using any cessation method or product. Quitting is just plain hard. Not only do you have to overcome your body's addiction to nicotine but you also need to attack the habit itself, that is, the behavioral structure you've developed to support your smoking. The most effective cessation methods address both addiction and habit.

You have to want to quit.

You can't quit smoking to please someone else, win a bet, or make a point. You have to want to stop. Without proper motivation, no cessation method in the world is going to work.

You have to be patient.

Few people make it on their first try. Backsliding isn't a sign of failure, just another step along the way. Don't use it as an excuse to avoid quitting.

You shouldn't go it alone.

You probably had a great deal of outside support when you started smoking. Since then you've no doubt built up quite a support system that encourages the habit (friends who smoke, favorite restaurants with smoking sections). Now that it's time to quit, you need to develop a support system for not smoking (friends who applaud your effort, restaurants where smoking isn't permitted).

There are also a number of not-for-profit and commercial programs available, such as:

• The American Cancer Society (ACS) has its own cessation program, Fresh Start, held in its local offices. The society also distributes information on smoking and smoking cessation. Contact the national office or check your local phone book for the nearest branch.

American Cancer Society
1599 Clifton Road, NE
Atlanta, GA 30329
(800) ACS-2345
http://www.cancer.org/tobacco.html

•Nicotine Anonymous is a twelve-step program modeled on
Alcoholics Anonymous. For literature, meeting schedules, or
other information, contact

Nicotine Anonymous World Services
PO Box 591777
San Francisco, CA 94159-1777
(415) 750-0328

•The American Lung Association offers its Freedom from
Smoking Clinic through local ALA offices. The association
also has a wide range of pamphlets ranging from tips for quitting tobacco to keeping a smoke-free home.

American Lung Association
1740 Broadway
New York, NY 10019
(212) 315-8700

•The Seventh-Day Adventists employ a spiritual approach to
quitting called the Breathe-Free Plan.

Seventh-Day Adventists
Narcotics Education, Inc.
12501 Old Columbia Pike
Silver Spring, MD 20904-1608
(800) 548-8700

You should consult with your doctor.

Although some nicotine replacement methods are now available in nonprescription form, you should consult your doctor before using any of them. In fact, your doctor should be part of the whole quitting process. Not only can your doctor recommend various methods and programs, and keep you informed about newer therapies, but also monitor your progress and illustrate for you how the benefits of not smoking are setting in.

Present drug therapies include nicotine chewing gum, transdermal nicotine patches, nicotine nasal spray, and nicotine inhalers. These nicotine replacement therapies wean you off the drug by gradually reducing your nicotine intake. Nicotine gum and patches are both available over-the-counter; nasal sprays and inhalers are, as of this writing, available by prescription only. A more recent therapy involves Wellbutrin, an antidepressant drug, which the FDA has recommended for use as a cessation therapy.

Although drug therapy may increase your chances of quitting, the most important factor remains motivation. If you don't *want* to quit, you may find yourself in the same spot as many dedicated smokers who end up using these products with, rather than instead of, cigarettes. That's not only counterproductive but dangerous as well; for example, more than a few smokers have brought on heart attacks by smoking in conjunction with a nicotine patch (another reason to have a doctor monitor your method and progress).

Nor should you rely upon drug therapies to handle your whole smoking problem. Drugs are best used in conjunction with a program that addresses the psychological, habitual side of smoking. After all, chewing gum is hardly an answer to

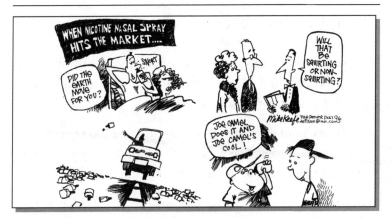

Mike Keefe/*The Denver Post*/diPIXion Studios, Inc.

that empty feeling you get every morning when you sit down with a cup of coffee and the newspaper. Here are some handy tips to help you or your kid get over cigarettes:

•When you quit, accentuate the change. Get rid of your smoking paraphernalia. Give away the ashtrays. Clean the house. Wash your clothes that smell like tobacco. Make a clean break and get a fresh start.

•You're probably used to hanging out where smoking is allowed (if not encouraged). Well, you're going to need some new hangouts. The good news is that now that you're a nonsmoker, you're not only welcome at far more public places but you're comfortable there as well.

•For the first few weeks you're going to be susceptible to backsliding, so avoid occasions that might tempt you. Avoid smoke and smokers for the time being.

•When you head into the movies (or watch one on television), be ready for the "Bogart effect": Everyone in the movie smokes and everyone looks so good doing it. You really miss smoking. When the movie ends, go for a brisk walk. Take deep breaths and remind yourself of the reasons you've decided to quit. Drink lots of water.

• Stay away from foods and drinks that remind you of cigarettes. If you're used to having a cigarette with your morning coffee, start drinking juice or water in the morning.

• If you can't sit still because you feel the need for a cigarette, drink a glass of water. Go for a walk. Take a few deep breaths.

• Slow down when you eat. A lot of smokers rush through their meals in order to get to that lovely postprandial smoke; now you have the time to enjoy what you eat. You'll soon find that the meal tastes better, too. Once you're done eating, don't sit back and wonder what's missing. Do something; take a walk.

• Reward yourself for not smoking. Set aside the money you'd spend on cigarettes, and either save it as a non-smoking investment or buy yourself a congratulatory present.

• Now that you're a healthy person, take up a healthy hobby. Start jogging, or even simply walking. Join a local basketball or softball league.

• Remember that showers quench cravings of *any* sort.

• Realize that the moment you stopped smoking you became a non-smoker. You don't need to put a year, month, or week behind you to qualify. The moment you put out that last cigarette, your body started its repair work. Give yourself a pat on the back.

RESOURCES

Whatever your political stand on smoking—from "all tobacco advertising should be banned" to "caveat emptor"—there's a smoking group to suit you, whether its focus is regulation and legislation, parents and communities, educational programs, prevention, intervention, or prestidigitation. Many of these groups have Web sites with activities, information, news updates, forums, polls, and chat rooms.

Action on Smoking and Health (ASH)
2013 H Street, NW, Washington, D.C. 20006
(202) 659-4310; URL: http://ash.org/ash/
ASH was formed in 1967 by Executive Director John F. Banzhaf III, who in 1966 petitioned the FCC to apply the Fairness Doctrine to cigarette commercials. As a result, TV stations were required to donate time for anti-smoking ads, which eventually led to the tobacco industry's accepting a ban on broadcast cigarette ads.

American Academy of Pediatrics
The Homer Building
601 13th Street NW, Washington, D.C. 20004
(800) 433-9016

American Cancer Society (ACS)
1599 Clifton Road, NE, Atlanta, GA 30329
(800) ACS-2345; Fax: (404) 248-1780
ACS, which provides information about smoking education, prevention, and cessation, sponsors the nationwide annual Great American Smokeout. For the local ACS office in your area, contact national headquarters or—for a little exercise—look it up in your neighborhood phone book.

American Heart Association (AHA) National Center
7272 Greenville Avenue, Dallas, TX 75231
(800) AHA-USA1

American Lung Association (ALA)
1740 Broadway, New York, NY 10019-4274
(212) 315-8700 or (800) LUNG-USA
ALA has more than 240 local offices in the United States; you can find the closest office by calling them at (800) LUNG-USA. The association, a leading source of information and education about lungs, is expert on the hazards of smoking. ALA also sponsors programs to quit smoking.

American Medical Association
515 North State Street, Chicago, IL 60610
(312) 464-5957

Americans for Non-Smokers Rights
2530 San Pablo Avenue, Suite J, Berkeley, CA 94702
(510) 841-3032; Fax: (510) 841-7702; URL: http://www.no-smoke.org

Centers for Disease Control and Prevention (CDC)
4770 Buford Highway, NE, Mail Stop K-50, Atlanta, GA 30341-3724
(800) CDC-1311

Coalition on Smoking or Health
1150 Connecticut Avenue, NW, Suite 820, Washington, D.C. 20036
Phone: (202) 452-1184; Fax: (202) 452-1417

Doctors Ought to Care (DOC)
561 S. Kirby Drive, Suite 440, Houston, TX 77005
(713) 798-7729 or (800) 362-9340
A not-for-profit organization founded in 1977, DOC is a leader in imaginative counteradvertising schemes that expose and ridicule tobacco and alcohol marketing.

National Cancer Institute
(800) 4-CANCER

National Center for Tobacco-Free Kids
1707 L Street, NW, Suite 800, Washington, D.C. 20036
(202) 296-5469; Fax: (202) 296-5427
The National Center for Tobacco-Free Kids runs the Campaign for Tobacco-Free Kids, which provides information and assistance to more than a hundred health, civic, and other groups dedicated to reducing tobacco use among America's children.

National Institutes of Health
National Institute on Drug Abuse
5600 Fishers Lane, Rockville, MD 20857
(800) 729-6686

Office on Smoking and Health (OSH)
National Center for Chronic Disease Prevention and Health Promotion (NCCDPHP)

Smoke-Free Class of 2000
7272 Greenville Avenue, Dallas, TX 75231-4596
(214) 706-1186; Fax: (214) 696-5211
The American Lung Association, American Cancer Society, and the American Heart Association together sponsor the Smoke-Free Class of 2000, so named for former Surgeon General C. Everett Koop's call for a smoke-free society by the year 2000. The program concentrates on graduating a smoke-free high school class in the year 2000, but the program is likely to continue into the following years.

Stop Teenage Addiction to Tobacco (STAT)
511 East Columbus Avenue, Springfield, MA 01105
(413) 732-7828; Fax: (413) 732-4219
STAT runs a national campaign to stop the sale of tobacco to children and teenagers. Members (dues start at $10) receive the group's quarterly newspaper, *The Tobacco-Free Youth Reporter.*

A FINAL THOUGHT

The tobacco war is still being waged—in the media, in congress, at the FDA, over the airwaves, in the schools, and in the homes. It it too dramatic to call it a war? Not when the number of deaths from smoking far outnumber military casualties caused by bombs and bullets. It is a high-stakes war involving both billions of dollars and the fate of a highly addictive drug. Despite news of possible settlements, it's not over yet.

New fronts are opening up. As a country we recognize the tremendous dangers and high costs of smoking. Therefore the tobacco industry is aiming their weapons at overseas markets. With fewer regulations, these cash-hungry governments may be eager enough for the short-term benefits of cigarette tax money to ignore the horrendous long-term costs of tobacco consumption.

Tobacco companies are currently pressuring congress to force other countries to accept tobacco or face economic retaliation from the U.S. This situation is similar to England forcing China to buy narcotics during the Opium Wars. If the U.S. continues to support the export of tobacco, future generations will look back on this time in our country with the same contempt.

If you are interested in the health of children worldwide, you must add your voice to those protesting the strong-arm sales of cigarettes overseas. Let's help parents worldwide do what we want to do: Raise smoke-free kids.